Smoking

Smoking

Making the Risky Decision

W. KIP VISCUSI

New York Oxford
OXFORD UNIVERSITY PRESS
1992

Oxford University Press

Oxford   New York   Toronto
Delhi   Bombay   Calcutta   Madras   Karachi
Kuala Lumpur   Singapore   Hong Kong   Tokyo
Nairobi   Dar es Salaam   Cape Town
Melbourne   Auckland

and associated companies in
Berlin   Ibadan

Library of Congress Cataloging-in-Publication Data
Viscusi, W. Kip.
Smoking : making the risky decision / W. Kip Viscusi.
p. cm.   Includes bibliographical references and index.
ISBN 0-19-507486-6
1. Smoking—United States—Psychological aspects.
2. Tobacco habit—United States—Psychological aspects.
3. Smoking—Economic aspects—United States.
4. Tobacco habit—Economic aspects—United States.
5. Decision-making—United States.
6. Risk-taking (Psychology)—United States.
I. Title.
HV5765.V57   1992
616.86'5—dc20   91-47138

9 8 7 6 5 4 3 2 1

Printed in the United States of America
on acid-free paper

Preface

Smoking has been a target of public health policies for several decades. Long before product risk regulation had become extensive, the government mandated hazard warnings for cigarettes, imposed restrictions on cigarette advertising, and engaged in an extensive informational campaign. More recently, restrictions on where these products can be consumed have also become widespread. The result has been a dramatic decrease in societal smoking rates. Whereas the majority of all adults once smoked, now fewer than three out of every ten American adults smoke, and this rate is continuing to decline. Cigarette smoking provides a large-scale natural experiment for assessing the impact and efficacy of government risk-communication efforts.

The focus of this book is on the character of the choice process that leads to smoking behavior. In particular, are smokers cognizant of the risks connected with smoking, and how do these risk beliefs influence the decision to smoke? Since these findings are likely to be of broad interest to researchers in a wide variety of fields as well as participants in the smoking policy debate, the text has been written in a manner that will make the results broadly accessible. Statistical and mathematical formulations are, for the most part, relegated to appendixes.

The overall theme of the book is that there have been a variety of sources of information provided to individuals about smoking risks, and the result is that perceptions of smoking hazards are substantial. In making judgments concerning the accuracy of risk perceptions, I take the risk assessments of the U.S. Surgeon General at face value. Thus, I do not question official risk assessments, but I focus instead on whether smokers are cognizant of the risks. Not only are these risk perceptions quite high, but they are also reflected in smokers' behavior.

The substantial awareness of smoking risks and individuals' response to them do not, however, imply that smoking decisions are ideal. Indeed, this research suggests that these decisions may be impeded by inaccurate risk perceptions. The observed biases and distortions in smoking decisions are not completely random, but are quite systematic. We can say a great deal about the kinds of mistakes people make and their causes. These shortcomings are pertinent both to the ongoing debate over smoking policy as well as to our understanding of how people grapple with the complex choices that may endanger their lives.

My interest in smoking is a natural extension of two decades of professional work on various aspects of health and safety risks. These studies have included examinations of the economic implications of job safety, product safety, and environmental risks. During the past decade much of my research has been concerned with the role of risk-communication efforts. The initial wave of government regulation in the 1970s adopted a technological approach to the promotion of health and safety. In the 1980s, there was an attempt to augment these policies by utilizing the capacity of individuals to influence the risks they face. Hazard-warning efforts proliferated as concern with individuals' right to know became a more prominent policy issue.

Cigarette smoking represents perhaps the ideal context for augmenting the experimental evidence on risk communication with results from an actual market experiment. The various waves of cigarette warnings and smoking information have played a particularly prominent role within the context of society's response to the risks of smoking. Moreover, the patterns of smoking behavior that result provide a rich context for assessing the implications of hazard communication for risk-taking behavior.

There are a variety of sources of information that we can use to analyze this behavior. Because of the long time frame over which this risk-communication activity has occurred, one obvious source of information is historical data. We can track smoking rates over time as well as the evolution of smoking risk perceptions. One can also analyze the relationship of smoking behavior to other risky choices. One such class of behavior that I will address here is how smoking behavior is linked to the risk-taking decisions of workers on the job.

During the course of my research on smoking risks, I was asked to share my expertise on risk perceptions and choice under uncertainty with Jones, Day, Reavis & Pogue, which is one of the law firms representing the cigarette industry. This effort never involved participation in any legal or regulatory proceeding. In the course of my discussions with them, I learned of a national survey that had been undertaken on their behalf to assess consumer attitudes and risk perceptions with respect to smoking. The survey design was quite sound, and the data represented a rich source of information for examining a variety of aspects of smoking behavior. These data, which I will refer to below as the Audits & Surveys data, will be a primary focal point of the empirical analysis in the book. I would particularly like to thank Barbara Kacir for calling these data to my attention and for many fruitful discussions of smoking issues.

To ensure the validity of the data, I also undertook a variety of sensitivity tests. The first was to replicate the exact survey question with a different sample. I also experimented with several other variants on the survey format to ensure the validity and robustness of the survey responses. All these efforts corroborated the survey results and extended the survey's focus to other measures of smoking risks.

I have included a copy of the text of the original survey in Appendix A. Readers wishing to validate the survey can readily do so with the aid of a telephone. In addition, in all class and seminar presentations of this research, I usually begin by eliciting the key survey responses from the audience, which almost invariably are strongly supportive of the survey results.*

---

*The main exception was an audience of students and faculty at the Stanford Risk Analysis Seminar. On the basis of a show of hands, participants in the seminar indicated their assessed risk level for cigarette smoking. Since students at the seminar could see the responses of two quite prominent and well-informed faculty members seated near the front—Kenneth Arrow and Amos Tversky—the clustering of responses near those of the above mentioned risk experts was not surprising.

My only direct work for the cigarette industry has been the assistance I gave to R. J. Reynolds with respect to the design of the hazard warning for the Premier cigarette. This cigarette involved a change in the cigarette technology that eliminated the burning of tobacco and also lowered some of the risk attributes of the product. My task was to assist in designing a warning that would convey the cigarette's fire-related hazards and the appropriate precautions.

The extensive research that I undertook for this book has not been supported either by the cigarette industry or by any law firms representing them. Moreover, even if this had been the case, I believe the results would stand on their own merits. I report extensive empirical tests and detailed information that will enable readers to make their own judgments regarding the validity of the empirical phenomena that I identify. Much of the study is based on either publicly available information or on data sets that are easy to replicate so that other researchers can readily validate the findings.

The rationale for drawing all this research together in a book form rather than a series of articles is that the evidence is much more compelling when viewed in its entirety than when considered on a piecemeal basis. I have given extensive presentations of this work at the Stanford University Risk Analysis Seminar, the Fifth International Conference on the Foundations of Decisions under Risk and Uncertainty, and at the American Economic Association meetings. The reception these groups have given to my work has been quite favorable. Comments by participants in these seminars have also led to numerous improvements in the analysis. I would also like to thank Duke University for providing me with a small grant to support this research.

Several individuals contributed to bringing this project to completion. At Oxford University Press, Herbert Addison and Mary Sutherland offered valuable advice and enthusiastic support. Sharon Tennyson and Patricia Born assisted with the computer programming, and Eric Ralph undertook the North Carolina phone survey. Lisa Larson handled everything else.

Portions of this book appeared previously as "Do Smokers Underestimate Risks?" *Journal of Political Economy* 98 no. 6 (1990), pp. 1253–1269; and "Age Variations in Risk Perceptions and Smoking Decisions," *Review of Economics and Statistics*, 73, no. 4 (1991), pp. 577–588.

Durham, N.C.   W. K. V.
February 1992

Contents

Smoking

1

Smoking as a Regulated Risky Decision

THE ECONOMIC SIGNIFICANCE OF SMOKING BEHAVIOR

Smoking risks arise from an individual's choice to engage in smoking behavior.[1] In contrast, many environmental and occupational hazards do not involve any market transaction and are completely involuntary in nature. Nuclear hazards and toxic wastes are two such risks.

In part because of this difference in character, smoking policies have not followed the pattern of other forms of risk regulation in terms of either their time frame or their structure. The decade of the 1970s marked a tremendous expansion in the scope of risk and environmental regulation. Congress created a variety of new federal agencies that adopted a myriad of technological standards to control risk. This surge in regulation was followed by a period of relative regulatory stagnancy in the early 1980s.

The pattern of regulation for smoking has been quite different. The government has never imposed specification standards regarding the design of safe cigarettes. In particular, the government has never mandated filters or particular cigarette designs in the same manner as it has attempted to alter the designs of risky consumer products and the technology of the nation's workplaces.

The emphasis instead has been on decreasing smoking activity rather than changing the safety properties of the product, whereas the dominant approach in government risk-regulation efforts over the past quarter century has been a technology-oriented focus. This emphasis of the cigarette risk-regulation efforts on altering behavior and providing information makes smoking the most well-developed case study for analyzing the efficacy of this regulatory approach.

As part of the social efforts to address smoking behavior, the government has initiated a broad array of policies. We have banned smoking ads on television and radio. Cigarette packages and advertising for cigarettes on billboards and in print must include hazard warnings. In addition, there is widespread publicity against smoking behavior led by government officials, including annual reports by the Surgeon General alerting the public to smoking hazards. Finally, there are a number of direct controls on smoking behavior at various government levels. These include local antismoking ordinances as well as national restrictions prohibiting smoking on airplanes.

Although fewer people smoke now than did in the past, many continue to smoke even in the presence of these antismoking efforts. A common belief is that individuals who smoke are ignorant of smoking's hazards and are incapable of making risky choices in a reliable manner. The evidence to be examined in this book suggests that we should abandon this stylized view. Instead of widespread ignorance of the risks, there is in fact substantial awareness of the potential hazards of smoking, even among smokers. The levels of awareness differ for various components of the risks of cigarettes. These perceptions reflect the influence of a complex mix of informational and cognitive factors. For example, the usual assumption by economists that extensive information leads to accurate risk beliefs is certainly not borne out.

There are also important manifestations of economic rationality. Higher assessed risks of smoking decrease individuals' willingness to smoke, as one would predict using a model of rational economic behavior. Substantial credit for creating these high risk perceptions should be given to government policy, which has contributed to the increase in risk perceptions over time.

The essential ingredient of smoking risks is that they arise from an individual product choice that potentially affects one's health. Individuals make a consumption decision about whether they will engage in smoking that is not entirely different from deciding on one's diet or new car purchase.[2] What we would like to know is the character of the choices that are made. What factors affect smoking decisions? Do individuals have an accurate sense of the potential hazards posed by smoking? Do they take these risks into account when making their smoking decisions? The answers to these questions affect the extent to which smokers are engaged in this behavior as the result of a deliberate choice. If smokers are unaware of the risk, for example, the existence of a market transaction to purchase cigarettes or other forms of tobacco would in no way imply that the risk-taking decision was voluntary.

In this book I will explore in detail the character of individuals' risk perceptions and the tradeoffs they make with respect to smoking. This assessment will include a variety of measures of smoking risk perceptions and the effect of these risk perceptions on smoking decisions. The fundamental issue is whether people understand and act upon the potential adverse effects of smoking behavior. This examination of smoking decisions is more extensive than any comparable individual choice analysis undertaken to date, whether it be the purchase of hazardous products or work on risky jobs.

PRINCIPAL FINDINGS

Assessing the adequacy of individuals' risk perceptions and smoking behavior necessarily entails that we utilize information based on these consumption decisions. Two classes of information potentially could be useful. First, we could assess how smoking patterns and public perception of smoking risks have changed in response to shifts in the information provided to the public about the hazards of smoking. Unfortunately, the temporal changes in smoking policies have not been perfectly controlled experiments. A variety of policy shifts have often occurred simultaneously, making it difficult to distinguish the separate influences at work.

Although we will draw upon this historical information in assessing smoking behavior, the focal point of the book will be on new sets of survey data that provide explicit information on individuals' risk perceptions and smoking behavior. Gathering data on an individual basis enables us to assess individuals' perception of the hazards of smoking and the effect of these risk perceptions on their decisions, which is the main matter of interest.

Utilization of original survey data also enables us to address a variety of concerns that could not even be raised using market-based data. For example, are smoking risk perceptions too high or too low? How does the accuracy of these risk perceptions vary with the particular type of smoking risk and the publicity it has received? Do individuals integrate these risk perceptions in their smoking decisions? How do risk perceptions regarding smoking relate to the information that individuals may have heard about cigarettes and their overall reactions to cigarettes as a product? The data sets we will examine provide detailed information that will enable us to better understand the smoking decision and this important class of consumer choices under uncertainty.

Summary of Results

The book begins with an assessment of the issues involved in the learning and risk-perception portions of the decision process. What are the sources of risk information, and how are they utilized in forming risk perceptions?

Chapter 2 considers how people make decisions under uncertainty generally and then relates these properties to smoking behavior.

Three different models of individual decisions are distinguished. First, smokers may be fully rational in terms of their risk perceptions and subsequent decisions. This approach is the standard economic model of fully informed choice. The second model is what is termed the "stylized smoker," which is the main characterization of smokers underlying the smoking debate. The stylized smoker is not aware of the risk and, if the risk is perceived, does not act upon this information in a sensible manner. The final possibility is that of a smoker who has cognitive limitations. It is this individual who acts in a manner that is consistent with the literature documenting a variety of systematic biases and errors in choices under uncertainty.[3] The thrust of the evidence presented in subsequent chapters will support the cognitive limitations model, although these limitations affect a choice process that is in many ways quite reasonable.

A variety of biases have been identified in the risk and uncertainty literature, including an overreaction to salient events and low probability outcomes. Because of the diversity of these biases and the multi-attribute character of smoking risks, there are no clear-cut predictions regarding the direction of smoking decision errors that one can generate based on this literature. We know how specific factors affect risk perceptions, but risk beliefs that are subject to a myriad of influences with conflicting effects are more difficult to predict. Smoking hazards are among the most prominent risks in society, and this aspect of smoking will play a central role in governing the societal response.

One of the most important potential contributors to smoking risk perceptions is the information provided to consumers about the potential hazards of smoking. This information has included government reports on smoking risks that have appeared on almost an annual basis for over two decades, as well as a series of smoking warnings, newspaper and magazine articles about smoking risks, and mentions of smoking hazards in cigarette advertising. Chapter 2 also documents the extent of this information and the long history of availability of smoking risk information. Although there is evidence of increased prominence being given to the risks of smoking, the dissemination of smoking information should not be regarded as either a recent phenomenon or one that depends solely on the emergence of government policy. Even before the government research reports and various regulatory actions against cigarettes, health hazards of smoking were prominently featured in the media and in cigarette advertising.

Ideally, warnings for cigarettes should lead individuals to form an accurate assessment of the risk based on these warnings. In the case of the 1965 warning, respondents believed that the warning implies a lifetime cancer risk of .12—a figure that is roughly of the same order of magnitude as the estimated lifetime cancer risk posed by cigarettes. Although there is no claim of pinpoint accuracy with respect to the precision of the risk information conveyed, the fact that such a subjectively worded and succinct warning could convey a risk level that is even of a reasonable order of magnitude is quite striking indeed. Individuals might, for example, have concluded that the warning implied a risk level of 1/250, which is comparable to the lifetime risk of death on a typical blue-collar job, or 1/3,000, which is the lifetime risk of fatality in an airplane crash.

There has been at least some public perception of smoking hazards for decades, if not for centuries. Review of the public opinion poll data in Chapter 3 indicates a belief that smoking is risky for as long as U.S. public opinion polls on smoking have been taken. The extent and diversity of the perceptions of risks have also increased over time.

Perhaps the greatest change in public attitudes toward smoking has been with respect to the public's willingness to take actions to restrict smoking behavior. In earlier decades there was substantial reluctance to advocate restrictions on smoking in public places. By the 1980s enthusiasm for such policies became widespread, and by the 1990s this support had led to smoking restrictions in almost every locale, including the major tobacco-producing states. This shift in attitudes may be influenced by factors other than altered risk perceptions. Imposing smoking restrictions has also become more acceptable politically, as the fraction of the U.S. population of smokers has diminished to about one-third.[4]

Examination of the trends in smoking risk perceptions in Chapter 3 illuminates the public's growing awareness of the potential risks of smoking, but it does not enable us to determine whether the risk assessments are too high or too low. The fact that people are aware of a particular risk does not necessarily indicate that the level of the risk perceived is correct.

In Chapter 4 I provide results from several surveys, including a large-scale national survey of lung cancer risk perceptions. The participants in that survey indicated the number out of 100 smokers who would develop lung cancer, where these responses and other survey information are used to explore the character of individual risk perceptions.

The main finding with respect to risk perceptions for lung cancer is that not only is there substantial awareness of the smoking hazards, but overall individuals appear to overestimate the risks as compared with the levels in the scientific evidence. Whereas the best scientific estimates of the lifetime lung cancer risks from smoking range from .05 to .10, individual perceptions of the risk are much greater. The entire population assesses this risk at .43, and even current smokers have a substantial risk perception of .37. The fraction of the population under-assessing the risk is less than 10 percent, and the extent of their risk underestimation is comparatively small in magnitude.

This pattern of overestimation may surprise many participants in the smoking debate, but it is quite consistent with other evidence on highly publicized hazards. People frequently overassess widely publicized risks, whether the risks are those of smoking or the chance of being killed by lightning or a tornado. One contributor to this overassessment of the risk is that these public accounts call individuals' attention to the adverse outcome but do not indicate the probability that the event will occur. Media accounts provide frequent and selective coverage of the numerator of the risk (e.g., the number of tornado deaths) without information on the denominator (e.g., the size of the reference population), making incorporation of public information into risk judgments difficult. The annual reports of the Surgeon General have a similar emphasis on tallies of the adverse health outcome without indicating the number of smokers or the intensity of the product's use.

Since the lung cancer risk has long been the most highly publicized smoking hazard, one would expect it to be the most prone to overestimation. The new survey data presented in Chapter 4 indicate that there is less of a tendency to overestimate the total mortality risk of smoking or the adverse effect of smoking on life expectancy, although these are overestimated somewhat as well. What is especially noteworthy is that for the different classes of smoking risks the amount of information provided increases rather than eliminates the bias in risk assessment. The most publicized smoking risks—lung cancer hazards—tend to be overestimated more than less-publicized components of the risk. This result is contrary to standard economic models of information provision. This anomalous result can be traced to the aforementioned character of the risk information provided.

This risk-perception bias finding also directly contradicts the stylized smoker model that generally serves as the backdrop for current social debate over smoking behavior. The potential for risk overestimation is not entirely surprising. The social controversy over the desirability of smoking has also created substantial public awareness of the potential risks of smoking. This controversy has apparently dominated the favorable influence of substantial cigarette advertising, which continues at a level of $1 billion per year.[5] A failure to incorporate such highly publicized information in forming one's risk perceptions would require that only the leading participants in the smoking debate are aware of the risk issues, not the public at large. The health outcomes associated with smoking are not hidden risks but instead have been the object of prominent public discussion for decades. For people to be completely uninformed about these potential risks would require a degree of ignorance that exceeds any shortcomings in individual behavior that have ever been documented in the literature. The evidence of high risk perceptions is consequently not surprising but is exactly what one would expect given the character of the information that has been provided as well as the extent of the antismoking efforts.

Examination of smoking risk perceptions also enables us to explore the nature of the learning process. The substantial precision of smoking risk judgments is reflected in the fact that many informational variables pertaining to ideas that the individual may have heard about smoking, such as whether smoking is hazardous to one's health, have no significant effect on smoking risk perceptions. Individuals who have heard that smoking is dangerous are likely to have risk assessments comparable to those who have not heard such claims. This type of phenomenon would not be the case for a product with hidden risks that must be called to consumers' attention before there is some realization of a potential hazard. The substantial invariance of smoking risk perceptions to a variety of background information questions suggests that individuals have highly developed smoking risk perceptions based on a very strong information base. The precision of the risk perceptions does not necessarily imply that these assessments are accurate, only that people are utilizing a wealth of information in forming their risk judgments.

Even if smoking risk perceptions are high, the key economic question is whether people act upon these risk perceptions in making their smoking decisions. Risk taking is an inescapable feature of our lives. The U.S. Department of Transportation estimates that the increased reliance on small, fuel-efficient cars in the 1980s has led to an additional 1,300 deaths annually, as consumers trade off higher fatality risks for greater fuel efficiency.[6] What we find in Chapter 5 is that smokers make similar tradeoffs. Changes in the tradeoff rate arising from a higher assessed risk of smoking exert a statistically significant and substantial effect on the likelihood of smoking.

The extent of the effect is reflected by how smoking behavior would change if people had accurate lung cancer risk perceptions. People are more likely to overestimate than underestimate this risk component of smoking. More importantly, because of the comparatively low level of the risk, the extent of the risk overassessment is much greater than the extent of the underassessment. The empirical results imply that if people had accurate perceptions of the lung cancer risks linked to smoking, then societal smoking rates would rise by 8 percentage points. For this national sample, the fraction of smokers would consequently increase from about one-third to two-fifths of the adult population.

The fact that smoking rates would increase if society had more accurate lung cancer risk perceptions does not imply that more people should smoke or that nonsmoking readers of these findings should reconsider their nonsmoker status. Statements such as these involve normative judgments most economists would regard as inappropriate. Risks other than lung cancer are important as well. Moreover, any policy judgment about the optimal societal level of smoking requires an analysis with a different emphasis than what I have undertaken here, including full recognition of the societal effects of smoking. The market response to more accurate risk perceptions should properly be regarded as an index of the extent of the role of risk perceptions as well as an index of how the market would respond if risk perceptions were altered.

Government policies affecting smoking have included not only actions intended to influence risk perceptions and smoking behavior directly but also excise taxes. By raising the effective price of cigarettes, excise taxes will discourage smoking behavior in much the same manner as would higher risk perceptions. The impetus for taxes on smoking and alcohol, which are often labeled "sin taxes," has never been formal economic models of optimal taxation of risky commodities. Rather, legislators see the taxation of various luxury products as an important source of tax revenues. Most recently, they imposed taxes on yachts and on cars with a price tag above $30,000. The taxation of alcohol and tobacco has selected religious appeal as well.

From a public policy standpoint, what we would like to do is set the tax level for any commodity sufficient to lead product purchasers to internalize all the costs associated with the product and to make efficient choices. Assessing the costs to nonsmokers that must be covered by a tax is difficult. Smoking has complex effects, reducing the ultimate pension and social security costs imposed by smokers but raising the expected society's health insurance costs. Some of these costs are internalized at least in part, as in the case of health insurance premiums that vary with smoking status. The extent of the cost imposed on nonsmokers also must be taken into account, but here the evidence is even more imprecise.

As a result, I will focus on the optimal taxation from the standpoint of the individual risk-taking decision, which is the main focus of this volume. In particular, to what extent do excise taxes endow people with the equivalent of accurate risk perceptions? The underlying economic principle is that risk perceptions discourage smoking to a particular degree, and if there were no awareness of the risks of smoking we would like the excise tax to establish the appropriate discouragement of smoking. To the extent that individuals overassess the risk of smoking, excise taxes are not needed to fulfill this function for the average consumer. Excise taxes will, however, serve to endow people who have no risk awareness with some economic equivalent of a risk perception. By examining the risk equivalent generated by excise taxes we can obtain another perspective on the relative effect on smoking of excise taxes as compared with risk perceptions.

Excise taxes are in fact quite powerful. Cigarette excise taxes are tantamount to endowing people with substantial risk perceptions. The role of these taxes is equivalent to increasing lung cancer risk perceptions by roughly 50 percent of their current levels. Since smoking risk perceptions are already quite high, the net effect is that both the individuals' risk perceptions and the considerable excise taxes on cigarettes greatly discourage smoking behavior.

The decision to smoke cigarettes is not simply one of risk perceptions but also one of tastes.[7] In particular, individuals are willing to trade off the risk of smoking for other valued attributes of the product, notably the pleasure derived from cigarettes. If smokers do in fact differ from nonsmokers in a systematic way, one might expect to observe other differences in behavior as well. Smokers should be attracted to other risky pursuits if it is a willingness to bear risks that influences smoking behavior.

An examination of the labor market behavior of different groups indicates that there are in fact such predictable variations. Smokers are much more willing to accept work on a hazardous job than are nonsmokers. More specifically, the rate of compensation they require for the risks they must bear on risky jobs is less. This finding is not unique to smokers. People who choose not to wear seat belts are also more willing to work on a hazardous job. For the group of the population who both smoke and choose not to wear seat belts, the willingness to work on hazardous jobs is the greatest.

Consistency of such decisions across different classes of risk-taking activity does not in and of itself imply rationality. People could be making the same kinds of mistakes in different contexts. However, it does provide a consistency check on the smoking results.

The smoking decisions of the young are of particular interest because of the concern with the difficulty of quitting smoking. Chapter 6 focuses on this pivotal policy concern, which is the extent to which individuals are making rational decisions at the onset of their smoking consumption activity. It is the rationality of the choices of the younger portion of the sample that is especially relevant. Younger smokers are more likely to have higher risk perceptions than are older smokers, in large part because their mix of smoking information is different. Individuals in the younger age-groups draw upon a larger proportion of smoking risk information generated in the recent era of vigorous antismoking efforts.

One might have expected evidence indicating that the younger smoker groups would be less responsible. Teenagers, for example, are the main contributors to drunken driving risks on the highways as well as to a variety of other forms of accidents. Critics of the cigarette industry frequently charge that the objective of the companies is to lure younger people into smoking at an early age, before they are able to make sound decisions with respect to their future health, and then trap them into a smoking habit from which they cannot extricate themselves. The support for this highly stylized view is bolstered by references to behavior such as the aforementioned rate of teenage highway fatalities that are all too familiar to parents who have sought to purchase automobile insurance for their male teenage sons.

The results in Chapter 6 indicate that this stylized profile is more myth than reality. In the context of smoking there is not only substantial evidence of risk perceptions on the part of these younger groups but also an incorporation of these risk perceptions in the decision-making process in a manner similar to that of other age-groups. Indeed, the smoking rates of younger individuals are just as sensitive to risk perceptions as are those of older population groups.

Teenagers do not make sensible smoking decisions simply as a matter of chance. Smoking behavior is strongly influenced by risk perceptions, which will be based on the set of information that the individuals have about smoking. As the criticism of smoking has become more widespread and the warnings concerning the potential hazards have proliferated, the mix of information that younger consumers have about smoking implies a greater risk than does the information set possessed by older consumers. The higher risk perceptions of younger consumers do not necessarily reflect more reasonable or more responsible behavior than that of their elders. Indeed, the results indicate that the behavior of the younger cohorts, given any particular level of risk perceptions, is no different than that of the older age-groups. What differs is the character of the risk perceptions, which can be traced to the different informational environments in which these individuals have lived.

The rationality of smoking behavior has come into question with respect to the entire debate concerning addiction—a problem the Surgeon General had formerly labeled "habituation." There are clearly costs of change associated with smoking behavior. The fact that quitting smoking is even an issue implies the presence of some adjustment costs.

Irrespective of the medical designation of these costs, what matters from an economic standpoint are the following classes of issues. First, at the time when individuals initiate their smoking activity, do they understand the consequences of their actions and make rational decisions? Recent economic literature has suggested that addictions of various kinds might be rational, and it is this test of rationality that is most important when making any policy judgments with respect to it. We make choices throughout our lives that are costly to reverse—getting married, choosing a profession, selecting a place to live, and purchasing a car. The fact that reversing such decisions is costly does not imply that the choices are incorrect. Rather, we must be cognizant of the potential losses from mistakes when decisions are hard to alter. What we should try to ascertain is the extent to which individuals are making irrational choices and the extent of the losses that result. The findings of this study assist in illuminating the elements of this debate but are not intended to resolve it.

If we exclude the role of addiction and secondhand smoke, smoking can be characterized as an individual risk-taking activity. If these choices are informed and have no adverse effects on society, there would be no efficiency rationale for regulating this behavior.

A useful test of this economic approach is to ask whether we could make similar arguments on behalf of legalization of crack cocaine and other drugs. Two distinctions appear most salient. Smokers do not inflict substantial harm on society through crime and other antisocial behavior. A smoker who is out of cigarettes may attempt to "bum" a cigarette from a stranger who is a smoker, but he will not smash your car window and rip out your CD player to get money to support his habit. Second, smokers continue to function as normal productive members of society. Smoking does not interfere with their work. There is no smoking-related counterpart to drunken driving. Unlike subway engineers on cocaine who crash their trains or the allegedly drunken captain of the Exxon *Valdez*, drivers who smoke are not accident-prone. Most of the costs and benefits of smoking are borne by the smoker. The fundamental policy concern is whether these individual decisions are sound.

Even if we were to conclude that this form of risk taking is informed, this result is quite different from claiming that choices are in any way commendable or that they are the decisions we would make given our own preferences. However, the appropriate individual rationality test is whether individuals are incorporating the available information about smoking risks and are making sound decisions, given their own preferences, not our preferences or some social planner's notion of what these preferences should be.

THE DECISION CONTEXT OF THE RESULTS

Consideration of the principal findings of the book within the context of the structure of the smoking decision is the most coherent way to organize these results. Figure 1–1 indicates the nature of the factors that affect smoking and the pertinent linkages involved. The two inputs to the risk beliefs that individuals have about smoking are their own prior beliefs and the various kinds of risk information they have received. This information includes cigarette warnings, information provided by the media, cigarette advertising, experiences of other smokers, as well as information provided by the government. As is indicated in the sources of information section of Figure 1–1, the reference point that will be used as the incremental lifetime probability of lung cancer for a smoker is a range from .05 to .10. This range provides the risk assessments one would make based on processing of the information provided by the government. Similar reference points will be employed for the overall smoking mortality risk and the effect of smoking on life expectancy.

The private and public sources of risk information affect the posterior risk assessments shown on the right side of Figure 1–1, leading to an overall lung cancer risk assessment of .43 for the entire sample and .37 for smokers. In conjunction with the risk perceptions, individuals also use their assessment of the consumptive benefits that will be derived from smoking in making their smoking decisions. These benefits will depend on the mix of smoking products. Advertising for cigarettes also appears to be a potential influence, although economists generally view tastes as being inherent to the individual rather than being molded by advertising. What advertising does is to provide information about products to affect brand choice. The main economic influence affecting decisions consequently will be the mix of products that are offered to consumers. The price of these products will reflect the companies' marketing decisions and the magnitude of cigarette taxes. These excise taxes average 30.8 percent of retail cigarette prices in the year of the main survey considered in this study.

The combined effect of risk perceptions, the smoking product mix, and excise taxes will determine the expected utility that individuals derive from smoking

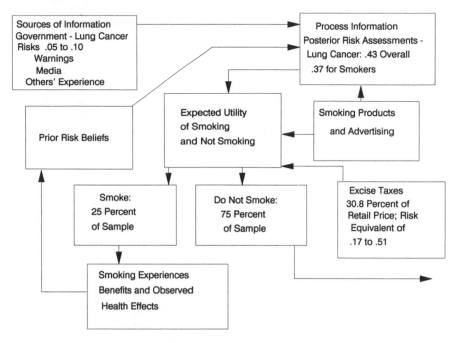

Figure 1–1 Structure of the smoking decision

behavior. Individuals for whom this expected utility exceeds that from not smoking will choose to smoke, as do 25 percent of the subjects in our national sample. Smoking behavior gives individuals information about the benefits to them of smoking as a consumption activity as well as feedback about possible observed health effects. These immediate effects can include coughing and shortness of breath, which are signals of a larger health risk that will influence perceptions of other risks. This information base then influences risk perceptions with respect to subsequent smoking behavior. As Figure 1–1 indicates, smokers are engaged in an ongoing process of making sequential decisions under uncertainty in a context in which there is a continuing flow of information from public sources and from the smoker's own experiences.

The overall picture that emerges is one of a class of consumption decisions that reflect the social controversy over smoking. When consumers are asked their opinion of cigarettes, their first reactions are almost invariably negative. They reply that smoking causes cancer, that smokers are idiots, or make some other unfavorable mention of cigarettes. Even smokers typically mention negative attributes of the product as a salient characteristic. The evidence is quite strong that there is an awareness of the potential risks of smoking as well as a substantial impact of these perceptions on consumption behavior.

The observed departures from the rational smoker model do not reflect individual irrationality so much as the character of reasonable individual responses in a highly imperfect informational environment. The informational campaigns emphasize the presence of a risk, not its magnitude. Substantial publicity given to a risk generally boosts perceptions of it, and smoking is no exception.

The implications of these results have far-reaching effects for smoking policies and risk-communication efforts more generally. Given this substantial smoking risk awareness, what is the appropriate role of the government with respect to these risky consumption decisions? Ideally, the objective of risk-communication efforts should be to foster informed choice so that individuals can make sound decisions cognizant of the risks generated by these actions. We do not wish to alarm individuals needlessly. Nor do we wish to lull them into complacency. The objective is not to alter behavior but to enable people to make the decisions that best advance their interests given the true properties of the actions they undertake.

What we find in the case of smoking is that risk perceptions are already quite substantial and perhaps even too high, particularly in the case of lung cancer. The findings in this book suggest that there should be a reassessment of the fundamental objective of smoking policies. The policy task should be redefined. Rather than simply discouraging smoking, our objective should be to foster more responsible risk-bearing decisions.

The proposed reorientation of the smoking policy efforts will not entail an abandonment of the government's role but rather will shift the emphasis toward efforts such as the promotion of safety through market competition. Despite the widespread awareness of smoking risks, there has been little policy effort to move to the next level of information refinement in which we communicate the risk differences among brands. These differences are not well understood. Moreover, present government policies do not promote innovation and competition with respect to cigarette safety. By adopting a policy approach that utilizes the choice process to promote market competition for safer cigarettes, we could better foster individual health and welfare.

NOTES

1. The focus here is on risks to the smoker. Secondhand smoke is one exception, as it clearly represents an externality that will not be fully addressed through decentralized choices.

2. Addiction issues are not raised with respect to cars, but they are for diet.

3. See, among others, the collection of papers in Kahneman, Slovic, and Tversky (1982). The academic journals *Journal of Risk and Uncertainty* and *Theory and Decision* are also devoted to these issues.

4. It should also be noted that with respect to these debates over competing "rights" to smoke or not to smoke, most economists would not even pose the issue in this manner. Assignment of property rights is of consequence if we are concerned with compensation. In this instance, however, compensation is not an issue. What we are seeking is an efficient outcome, not the preservation of assigned rights in a situation in which there is no market exchange. Determining the optimal smoking "rights" outcome involves establishing the benefits and costs of different forms of restrictions. This approach takes the problem out of its more strident and inconclusive ideological context in which the debate

has been waged. One must, however, still be concerned with the value of uncompensated losses.

5. U.S. Department of Health and Human Services (1989), p. 499.

6. *Product Safety and Liability Reporter* 18, no. 38 (1990), p. 1055.

7. The role of heterogeneity with respect to the value of health is a central theme in the health economics literature. See Fuchs (1986) and Manning et al. (1991).

2

The Cognitive and Informational Context

There have been two aspects of the policy debate over cigarette smoking. The first pertains to the risks posed by cigarettes. The potential hazards of smoking have been widely discussed in the media and in various government reports.

From the standpoint of potential market failures, the main issue is not whether there are potential risks of smoking—a relationship that is quite well known and in little dispute—but rather whether individuals who take these risks are cognizant of the possible hazards they face. The preponderance of the risks of smoking—roughly nine out of every ten smoking-related deaths—are borne by the smokers themselves.[1] From an economic standpoint, the fundamental issue is whether these hazards are well understood and whether the decisions people make with respect to these risks are rational.

The perceptions of the hazards of secondary smoke are of less consequence to assessments of the adequacy of information for individual decisions since these risks represent an involuntary externality. Smokers may take some of these risks into account, particularly for family members, but are not likely to undertake actions that are fully optimal from a societal perspective. An obvious potential market failure exists for secondary smoke irrespective of the smoker's risk perceptions. In contrast, market processes can lead to efficient risk levels for smokers if their consumption decisions are informed and rational.

The second major behavioral aspect of smoking pertains to the costs of altering smoking decisions. These costs were originally labeled a problem of "habituation" by the Surgeon General of the United States, who declared: "The tobacco habit should be characterized as an habituation rather than an addiction."[2] Based on more recent medical evidence regarding the health effects of smoking, former Surgeon General C. Everett Koop designated the problem as one of "addiction."[3] The average nicotine content of cigarettes has declined since the original habituation designation,[4] but the addictive characterization has become more stringent.

Irrespective of the label applied to the cost of altering cigarette smoking behavior, or whether one believes that cigarettes belong in the same category as crack cocaine and heroin, it is clear that cessation of smoking does involve real and substantial costs. The presence of transactions costs of altering behavior is, however, not unique. Costs of change are present in other economic contexts, such as leaving one's job, changing housing location, or altering one's diet. A considerable literature has been devoted to analyzing the implications of these costs for social welfare.[5]

Although the smoking addiction literature has not explicitly addressed the risk-perception issue, these issues are closely linked. If individuals are fully cognizant of the potential risks of smoking at the time when they begin their smoking decisions, and if they fully anticipate the costs of changing this behavior, market outcomes will be efficient. In contrast, there will be a greater potential for social losses if individuals are ill informed about the risks of smoking, subsequently discover that their smoking behavior poses risks to their health, and are discouraged from altering their behavior by the transactions costs of change. The extent of any individual welfare loss from inadequate risk perceptions will depend in large part on whether smokers and, in particular, relatively new smokers, are aware of the potential risks associated with their consumption decisions.

This chapter will first address the cognitive factors that govern risk perceptions generally and that will be influential in the smoking context as well. To provide a reference point for the subsequent discussion, I will summarize the evolution of hazard-warning labels for cigarettes and address the extent of media coverage of smoking hazards. This review will indicate that for the past several decades smoking risks have had increasingly substantial prominence.

THE DEBATE OVER SMOKING BEHAVIOR

The most fundamental issues in the smoking policy debate hinge on the degree to which smokers are making rational decisions. Assessing the rationality of this behavior entails more than simply noting whether people generally seem to be acting sensibly. Casual judgments of this type more often than not consist of a researcher assessing whether such behavior is consistent with the researcher's own tastes and beliefs. Moreover, even if some departures from rationality are observed, there is more than one potential way in which deviations could occur. There are several frameworks one could apply to model aspects of smoking behavior, with each having different normative implications.

Table 2–1 provides a summary of three principal perspectives on smoking behavior that can be distinguished. The first considers smokers as fully rational decision makers. Such individuals will make decisions consistent with the standard assumptions in an idealized economics textbook model of consistent consumer choice. This individual is fully informed and makes rational decisions based on this information.

The second perspective one could take is what I term the "stylized smoker." Such smokers are generally unaware of the risks. Moreover, if they are cognizant of the hazards, they ignore these risks in making their decisions. Variants of this view of smokers are most often implicit in the smoking policy debate.

The final alternative listed in Table 2–1 is that of a smoker with cognitive limitations. Decisions under uncertainty are notoriously difficult, and economists and psychologists have identified a variety of shortcomings in such decisions. Although this literature has not been explicitly concerned with smoking behavior

Table 2–1 Alternative perspectives on smoking behavior

	Rational smoker	Stylized smoker	Smoker with cognitive limitations
Sources of risk information	Utilization of public and private risk information in a rational learning process	Excessive attention to exhortatory smoking advertising and systematic neglect of risk information	Reliance on recent and highly publicized risk information
Risk perceptions	Accurate risk perceptions in the limiting full-information case; overestimates small risks and underestimates large risks with less than full information	Underassesses smoking risks, possibly even setting the risks to themselves, as opposed to society at large, at zero	Systematic biases in risk perception depending on the character of the risk; overestimates likely for highly publicized risks
Recognition of tradeoffs in decision	Balances utility value of smoking against expected utility loss from adverse health effects; weights future outcomes consistently with other future effects and in recognition of prevailing interest rates	Either unaware of the risks so that there is no tradeoff or else suppress existence of tradeoff; myopic behavior neglects future consequences	Overreacts to new and highly publicized risks and to identified risks that create fear and dread, such as cancer
Efficiency properties of the smoking decision	Efficient risk level in full information case	Risk is too high compared with idealized efficient market	Nature of inefficiency depends on nature of risk; excessive risk response to highly publicized risks

to any substantial degree, one could apply the insights of this literature to smoking based on the nature of the risky decision context. This "cognitive limitations" model of smoking behavior incorporates recognition of the systematic shortcomings of decision making in the presence of uncertainty.

To see how the implications of each of these three frameworks differ, let us consider the key components of smoking behavior summarized in Table 2–1. The sources of information that individuals use in forming risk perceptions will differ depending on the analytic approach. In forming risk perceptions, the rational smoker will take into account all of the diverse forms of information available, including information provided by the government, stories in the news media, personal experiences with smoking, and similar inputs. Moreover, the rational smoker will incorporate this information in a systematic learning process that satisfies a series of well-defined consistency properties. The usual test that economists and decision theorists impose for rational learning is that the individual acts in a Bayesian manner. More specifically, do people form and update their subjective probability assessments in a manner consistent with the laws of probability, that is, in a manner consistent with Bayes' Theorem for the updating of probabilities.[6]

The stylized smoker also has access to this information, but this smoker pays excessive attention to the exhortatory effect of smoking advertising and ignores the adverse information about smoking. Often implicit in this framework is the consumer's use of some kind of selective filter in terms of the information that is acquired, as only the information about the attractive attributes of cigarette smoking is processed.

In contrast, the model of the smoker based on the literature dealing with the cognitive limitations of choice under uncertainty views humans as having limits with respect to their information-processing capabilities. They cannot acquire and comprehend all publicly available information. In this world in which information acquisition and processing are costly, people will place excessive reliance on recent events that are vivid in their memory and on highly publicized risks. For example, dramatic risks such as those posed by earthquakes and similar risks that receive widespread media coverage are more likely to be represented in the risk-information set than are risks that receive very little press coverage relative to their magnitude, such as the risk of strokes.[7]

The second component of the models summarized in Table 2–1 is the risk perceptions that result from this information processing. These beliefs will not necessarily be fully accurate even in the case of the rational smoker. A rational individual considering alternative risks might begin by setting the chance of such risks as being equal, and he will then alter these assessments by integrating the information that he has about each class of risks. It is only after information is acquired about the specific risks that one will begin to move toward the true probability. Because of this partial learning process, a rational but not fully informed learner will tend to overestimate small risks and underestimate larger risks in the absence of full information.[8] The rational learner will adjust probabilities toward their true values but will not reach these values if information is incomplete. However, if the information provided concerning a risk is quite extensive and if this information is accurate, one would expect the rational smoker to have accurate risk perceptions. Given the voluminous amount of information that has been provided about cigarettes, the limiting full-information case is a plausible reference point for the rational choice model. Since, however, cigarette companies often provide favorable information and the government and media generally provide unfavorable information about smoking, the net effect is unclear. The problem is that not all information provided accurately conveys the risk.

The stylized smoker not only applies a filter to the risk information he or she has acquired but also tends to ignore the risks for which information is received. Moreover, even if there is awareness of smoking risks in general, this smoker is usually assumed to underassess the smoking risks to him- or herself (i.e., the "it won't happen to me" phenomenon).[9]

The literature on the actual decision process with respect to uncertainty emphasizes the much more subtle and complex processes at work. Systematic biases in risk perceptions are prevalent, but these biases may be in either direction. Much depends upon the character of the risk. Individuals tend to overestimate small risks and underestimate larger risks. They similarly overestimate risks that have been highly publicized or that involve substantial fear and dread, such as the risk of cancer. In contrast, hidden risks or risks that have not been the object of substantial or recent publicity will tend to be underestimated.

The way in which these risk perceptions enter the decision processes indicated in the third row of Table 2–1 differs greatly across the three models of behavior. Within the context of a rational economic model, the individual undertakes a careful balancing of the competing health risks associated with smoking and the utility derived from smoking. Moreover, the weight that the individual places on the deferred health risks as compared with the present welfare benefits of smoking is consistent with other kinds of intertemporal decisions that the smoker makes. It will generally be rational to discount future impacts, placing a lower weight on one's future utility than on one's present utility. The same role that interest rates have in influencing the intertemporal terms of trade one will make with respect to current and future consumption of all kinds will also be reflected in the relative weights one places on the deferred health effects of smoking in comparison with the immediate welfare benefits.

In the extreme case of the stylized smoker, there is no tradeoff whatsoever. The smoker simply ignores the risk component since these risks are remote. In situations in which the risk component is recognized, the stylized smoker neglects the future health impact by placing an insufficient weight on the future welfare benefits.

Some observers have hypothesized that the neglect of the future risks arises through a process of cognitive dissonance as the consumer denies the importance of the future health impacts. The stylized smoker framework assumes that the consumer's weighing of the intertemporal effects is one of myopic behavior. Only the immediate gratification provided by cigarettes drives consumer behavior.

The framework of smokers with cognitive limitations portrays smokers as overreacting to the new and highly publicized risks when making their decisions. There are, of course, other biases in decisions that arise from the character of the choice process rather than from the influence of inadequate perceptions of the risk. For example, some studies suggest that individuals are more willing to take a chance at experiencing a large adverse outcome than to face the certainty of a less-severe adverse outcome.[10] However, most variations of such effects appear not to be of substantial pertinence within the smoking context.

The final component of Table 2–1 is a summary index of the rationality of smoking choices. The net effect of these various components of the decision process influences the nature of the efficiency outcome. The rational smoker model provides the efficient market reference point. Some individuals may rationally choose to smoke, but these decisions will be efficient because they will fully reflect a deliberate tradeoff between the benefits rational smokers derive from cigarette consumption and the expected health risks.

In contrast, the stylized smoker will be incurring an inefficiently high level of risk. People will smoke more often than they should, and more people will smoke than would smoke in a fully informed and rational world.

Under the final model of individuals with cognitive limitations, we cannot say in general how decisions will be biased with respect to the efficiency of the risk level. However, if the influence of the highly publicized aspect of the risk is dominant, it is likely that there will be excessive attention to the risk, leading to less smoking than would be observed if people fully understood the risks. Other attributes of the risk such as the tendency to underestimate large risks, may, of course, work in different directions. As a result, even if one accepts the implications of the substantial literature on the shortcomings of individual choice under uncertainty, one still must explore empirically the specific inadequacies of the risk-decision process for cigarette smokers to ascertain the net impact of these influences.

THE DETERMINANTS OF RISK PERCEPTIONS

Before considering the results concerning the perception of smoking risks, it is instructive to begin with a review of what we know already about the character of individual risk perceptions.[11] The rationale for examining previous findings is twofold. First, a better understanding of the nature of the main features of risk perceptions that have been displayed in past studies will better enable us to predict what patterns should be observed in the cigarette smoking context. Having an objective reference point is particularly important because of the emotionally charged nature of the public smoking debate. Second, examination of the literature will enable us to ascertain what new lessons we can draw regarding the character of risk perceptions and the role of public information in influencing these perceptions. The smoking information initiatives undertaken by the federal government represent a large-scale social experiment in the provision of information, and ideally we should attempt to glean as much as we can from the impact of this informational effort so as to better assess the desirability of future informational programs.

Patterns of Bias

Some unknown hazards are associated with no risk perceptions at all, and other risks may be overestimated or underestimated. It would be overly simplistic to conclude that individuals simply make mistakes as probability assessors and that they are completely irrational in their subsequent decisions under uncertainty. In particular, there is substantial evidence that although people make errors, these errors are often systematic. The focus here will be on the character of the systematic biases that have been observed and their possible relevance to smoking hazards.

The first characterization of risk perceptions pertains to the level of the risk. A number of studies of mortality risks beginning with the article by Lichtenstein et al. (1978) indicate that individuals tend to overestimate small-probability events and underestimate large-probability events. In particular, individuals overestimate risks such as the chance of dying in a tornado or being killed by botulism or a smallpox vaccination, whereas the truly substantial risks of death—such as the chance of dying of heart disease, stroke, or stomach cancer—tend to be under-estimated.

This overestimation of small risks and underestimation of large risks is not an artifact that arises from inexplicable cognitive failures. To see how such a relationship can arise, consider Figure 2–1. The horizontal axis provides the actual risk level, and the vertical axis indicates the public's perception of the risk. If perceptions are accurate, they will lie on the 45-degree line for which actual and perceived risks are equated.

Suppose that individuals begin with a situation of highly imperfect information in which they have no specific knowledge of the levels of various sources of risk. If all risks are assessed equally, the initial beliefs will lie along the horizontal line shown in Figure 2–1. In this situation of ignorance, low probabilities are over-assessed and high-probability risks are underestimated.

Now let individuals obtain information about the risk either from their own experiences or from publicly provided information. If this information is accurate, the curve characterizing individuals' probabilistic beliefs will move closer to the 45-degree line in Figure 2–1. Because individuals' beliefs are a weighted average of their prior beliefs and the risk information they have received, actual and perceived risks will not generally be the same. Equality will only be achieved when the risk information obtained is so extensive that it dominates the influence of individuals' own prior beliefs.

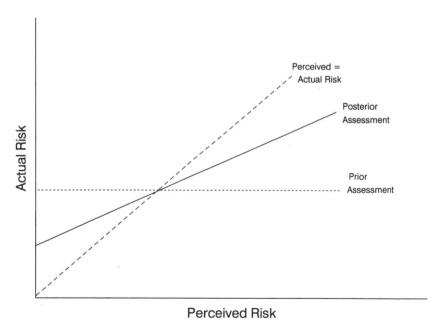

Figure 2–1 The nature of risk perceptions

The appropriate test of bias is whether the degree of learning toward the truth varies with the risk level. Using the original data developed by the psychologists who identified the risk-related bias phenomenon, I have shown that there is no significant relationship of the degree of learning with the level of the risk.[12] People learn about small and large risks to the same degree, but because this learning is partial, one finds the biases shown in Figure 2–1.

The pattern of risk perceptions is consistent with a rational learning process, but people lack full information. The absence of complete information accounts for the systematic biases that are observed. Equally important is that the size-related bias in risk perceptions is quite specific. Moreover, many of the other sources of bias to be cited below also are in a particular direction. The fact that there are departures from full rationality and an observed pattern of biases in perception does not imply that behavior is irrational, unpredictable, and erratic. The observed biases are quite systematic and can often be accounted for by a quite reasonable response to a world of highly imperfect information.

The implications of these risk-related bias results for smoking behavior are not entirely clear. Cigarette smoking risks over a lifetime are close to some of the extreme risk categories that have been examined in previous studies. As the risk breakdowns in Figure 2–2 indicate, the annual mortality risk that a smoker incurs from smoking behavior is much greater than that of many other common risky pursuits, such as operating a motor vehicle and job-related accidents. The incremental risk from cigarette smoking is, for example, larger than the average annual risk of dying of cancer—a large risk that tends to be underestimated.

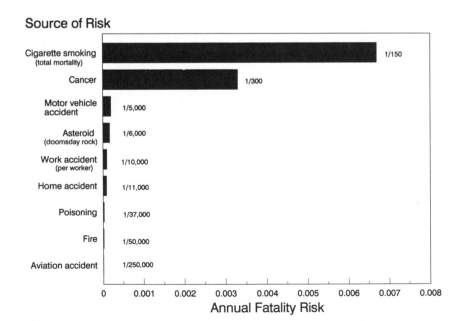

Figure 2–2   Comparison of different lifetime risks

Similarly, the risks of cigarettes are believed to be greater than the chance of being killed by a flood or some other very rare event, which are among the types of risks that are overestimated. On balance, the size of the lifetime smoking risk is sufficiently great that this influence should produce a tendency to underestimate the risk if it is the size of the lifetime risk that is the matter of concern.

The influence of the magnitude of the risk on the bias in risk perceptions also depends on the context in which the decision is framed. Lifetime risks are substantial, but the risks from a pack of cigarettes or a single cigarette are relatively small, producing a tendency to overestimate the risk level. An open issue that will affect the direction bias for smoking behavior is the extent to which individuals are thinking of the lifetime risk or the individual cigarette risk when making smoking decisions. Until this decision context issue is resolved, the predictions based on the size of risk bias is unclear.

Other biases in risk perception pertain to whether individuals have information about the risk and whether this information is salient. An early study of the risks of natural disasters by Kunreuther et al. (1978) indicated that people tended to ignore hidden low-probability events. In contrast, the risks from low-probability events that are called to peoples' attention are greatly overestimated, as found in the study by Viscusi and Magat (1987). Reconciling these conflicting studies in a consistent manner is possible by recognizing that hidden risks are underestimated, whereas small risks that are more prominent will tend to be overestimated. To the extent that cigarette smoking risks are among the most-discussed risks in our society, one would expect there to be an overestimation of these hazards.

This kind of effect is borne out most forcefully in studies that have explicitly examined the degree of publicity given to various hazards and the extent of the resulting biases in perception. The investigation of the assessed risks of mortality by Combs and Slovic (1979) and Slovic, Fischhoff, and Lichtenstein (1979) indicated that risks that have received the most media attention as measured by newspaper article coverage were the most prone to being overestimated. Given the prominent role of the cigarette smoking debate and the publicity given to cigarettes, smoking risks are clearly among the most highly publicized risks in our society. This set of influences would lead us to expect cigarette risks to be substantially overestimated.

This result contradicts the usual economic models of rational learning behavior. Should not more information about a risk lead risk perceptions to converge to the true risk value? This full-information result does not hold since newspaper stories and other publicity do not convey information regarding probabilities; rather, they focus on risk outcomes, which will raise the assessed frequency of the publicized adverse event.

The role of risk information and the extent to which one is an "informed" risk assessor is reflected in the risk perceptions of different classes of individuals. An interesting perspective on the potential biases in risk perception is obtained by comparing the view of risk experts with that of laypersons. The study by Slovic, Fischhoff, and Lichtenstein (1980a) considered the various relative risk assessments for thirty different accident groups. The task they gave the respondents was to rank the groups in order of the degree of mortality risk posed by the activity.[13]

The patterns shown in Table 2–2 indicate substantial variations in relative risk beliefs. College students and the League of Women Voters members ranked nuclear power risks as being the most substantial, whereas the experts ranked nuclear hazards as being twentieth among the thirty risk concerns. This difference reflects the apparent overestimation of the small but highly publicized risks of nuclear power.

The component of the table that is of greatest interest here is the assessment of smoking hazards. What is most striking is that in all the cases smoking risks are ranked among the top four perceived risks. The assessed risks from smoking exceed the perceived risks from police work, mountain climbing, and a wide variety of highly risky endeavors. In the absence of any information regarding

Table 2–2   Ordering of perceived risk for 30 activities and technologies

Activity	Experts	College students	Active club members	League of Women Voters
Motor vehicles	1	2	5	3
Smoking	2	4	3	4
Alcoholic beverages	3	6	7	5
Handguns	4	3	2	1
Surgery	5	10	11	9
Motorcycles	6	5	6	2
X rays	7	22	17	24
Pesticides	8	9	4	15
Electric power	9	18	19	19
Swimming	10	19	30	17
Contraceptives	11	20	9	22
General (private) aviation	12	7	15	11
Large construction	13	12	14	13
Food preservatives	14	25	12	28
Bicycles	15	16	24	14
Commercial aviation	16	17	16	18
Police work	17	8	8	7
Fire fighting	18	11	10	6
Railroads	19	24	23	20
Nuclear power	20	1	1	8
Food coloring	21	26	20	30
Home appliances	22	29	27	27
Hunting	23	13	18	10
Prescription antibiotics	24	28	21	26
Vaccinations	25	30	29	29
Spray cans	26	14	13	23
High school and college football	27	23	26	21
Power mowers	28	27	28	25
Mountain climbing	29	15	22	12
Skiing	30	21	25	16

Source: Slovic, Fischhoff, and Lichtenstein (1980a), p. 191.

% Who Believe Product Is Somewhat/Very Harmful

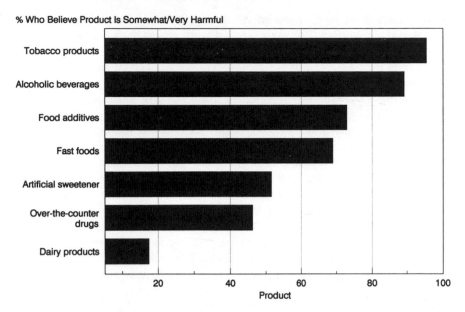

Figure 2–3 Public's belief in product riskiness. *Source:* U.S. Bureau of Alcohol, Tobacco, and Firearms, Final Report of the Research Study of Public Opinion Concerning Warning Labels on Containers of Alcoholic Beverages, December 1988, vol. 1, Table 2.

the quantitative scale represented by the rankings, these results do not indicate whether or not the risks of smoking are overestimated or underestimated by any of the four groups. Moreover, none of these results are adjusted to reflect the differing intensities of the activities. People smoke and ride in motor vehicles more often than they go mountain climbing, but this does not mean that mountain climbing is a safer pursuit. However, the results are suggestive of the overall prominence of smoking hazards in the public's perception. For all groups of individuals of varying informational backgrounds, smoking risk perceptions are among the highest of all the risky pursuits listed in Table 2–2.

The product risk belief comparisons in Figure 2–3 tell a similar story. Tobacco is considered to be more harmful than any other food or diet-related product, including alcoholic beverages and food additives. Indeed, nineteen out of every twenty respondents to this national survey undertaken for the U.S. Bureau of Alcohol, Tobacco, and Firearms viewed tobacco products as being "harmful" or "very harmful." This strongly negative view was expressed despite the presence of a large number of smokers among the respondents. In the subsequent sections, we will explore the evolution of these perceptions over time.

Hazard Warnings and Risk Perceptions

One mechanism for eliminating potential biases in risk perceptions is hazard warnings. Ideally, risk labeling efforts could communicate the hazards so that people can make a more informed risk-taking decision. The policy objective consequently is informed decisions coupled with consistent and rational choices under uncertainty.

Although there has been considerable recent literature on the impact of hazard warnings, the evidence pertaining to the accuracy of the risk perceptions resulting from these warnings is less complete. In a study of chemical labeling for workers, Viscusi and O'Connor (1984) showed that workers processed warning information in a manner that was consistent with a rational learning process.[14] In addition, the compensating wage differentials implied by these risk perceptions were consistent with the implicit values of injury in the literature on compensating wage differentials for risk. The strongest evidence in this study for the accuracy of risk perceptions was for workers who were in the warnings group for sodium bicarbonate. Working with household baking soda eliminates all disease risks for the job, leading workers to have risk perceptions identically equal to the acute accident probability for the chemical industry in which they worked.

Other evidence is consistent with a rational learning process but does not necessarily imply accurate perceptions. The studies of household chemical and pesticide warnings by Viscusi and Magat (1987) and Magat, Viscusi, and Huber (1988) indicate that there is consumer understanding of the warnings, an increase in risk perceptions resulting from the warnings, and an increase in precautionary behavior. While these studies suggest that warnings foster more accurate risk beliefs, these results do not imply that risk perceptions are ideal.[15]

The principal weak link is the character of the risk information provided. Hazard warnings are not tantamount to the provision of full and complete information. Rather, the typical warning alerts individuals to potential risks and the need for caution. The format, content, and amount of information are important matters of concern because of the limited information-processing capabilities of the recipients of the warnings. As a consequence, cigarette warnings quite correctly do not attempt to convey a detailed sense of the complex medical ramifications of smoking but instead have focused on a quite parsimonious message. Since 1984, cigarette packages and advertising have rotated four different short warnings, but this rotation means that any given warning will be seen only one-fourth of the time, thus diluting its impact.

When the succinct warning message is not wisely chosen, the effect may be worse than the loss from inadequate information. In some cases, the risk perceptions may be wildly out of line with the actual risks being conveyed. The pattern of risk perceptions arising from California's Proposition 65 (a food cancer risk-communication effort) indicates that the wording chosen for the cancer warning implies risk perceptions of 1/10—a level that exceeds the regulation's risk threshold for warning of 1/100,000 by a factor of 10,000.[16] In particular, this policy, which is not yet fully implemented, mandates a cancer-warning wording that is out of line with the trace levels of risk posed.

Although hazard warnings may communicate knowledge regarding the risk, the nature of the risk information conveyed is not precise. Hazard warnings typically indicate a danger and the associated precaution, but they seldom give exact probabilistic information regarding the health outcomes involved. A useful test of the degree to which individuals are accurately informed is to examine the explicit risk perceptions that result after the warnings are in place. This test will be the focus of Chapter 3. The main objective of this chapter will be to track the evolution of smoking risk perceptions.

SOURCES OF RISK INFORMATION

Although most smokers are not scientists or physicians, they nevertheless have considerable sources of information that they can and do use to form their judgments regarding the level and severity of possible smoking risks. One source of information is general societal knowledge, ranging from children being told that smoking will stunt their growth to more sophisticated discussions of the potential health hazards.

A second source of information is the direct experience of the smoker and the observation of experiences of other smokers. Many of the health effects, such as coughing and shortness of breath when exercising, are apparent. The morbidity effects are more immediate than the mortality effects, and they provide signals of the overall riskiness of smoking behavior.

A third source of information is that provided by the cigarette industry. That information, including advertising and other public relations efforts, will tend to foster a positive view of smoking.

Government Provision of Information

The fourth source of information most readily manipulated as a policy variable is that provided by the government. This information provision takes two forms. The government periodically issues reports on smoking behavior. In 1964 the government issued a landmark report on cigarette smoking that attracted widespread attention,[17] and for the last two decades, the Surgeon General has issued regular reports on the hazards of smoking.[18] The issuance of these reports is generally accompanied by a press conference that usually receives substantial media coverage.

Table 2–3 provides a summary of the report topics. Several features of this summary are most striking. First, the Surgeon General's public information reports have been a substantial and ongoing effort. Second, the diversity of risks treated by the reports has been quite extensive. Although many of the reports have had a general risk focus, others have addressed specific classes of risk, such as those pertaining to lung cancer and heart disease. The shift to reports with a narrowly focused theme may have stemmed in part from the greater media attention given to specific report findings rather than more broadly based risk overviews. The press can deal more readily with a single theme than with a comprehensive and more diffuse assessment of smoking risks. Although the broadly based 1964 report also attracted substantial attention, its main message

Table 2–3   The Surgeon General's reports on smoking

1967	The Health Consequences of Smoking: A Public Health Service Review
1968	Supplement to the 1967 Public Health Service Review
1969	Supplement to the 1967 Public Health Service Review
1970	No Report
1971	The Health Consequences of Smoking
1972	The Health Consequences of Smoking
1973	The Health Consequences of Smoking
1974	The Health Consequences of Smoking
1975	The Health Consequences of Smoking
1976	The Health Consequences of Smoking: Selected Chapters from the 1971–1975 Reports
1977–1978	(one edition) The Health Consequences of Smoking
1979	Smoking and Health —The Health Consequences of Smoking —The Behavioral Aspects of Smoking —Education and Prevention
1980	The Health Consequences of Smoking for Women
1981	The Health Consequences of Smoking: The Changing Cigarette
1982	The Health Consequences of Smoking: Cancer
1983	The Health Consequences of Smoking: Cardiovascular Disease
1984	The Health Consequences of Smoking: Chronic Obstructive Lung Disease
1985	The Health Consequences of Smoking: Cancer and Chronic Lung Disease in the Workplace
1986	The Health Consequences of Involuntary Smoking
1987	No Report
1988	The Health Consequences of Smoking: Nicotine Addiction
1989	Reducing the Health Consequences of Smoking: 25 Years of Progress
1990	The Health Benefits of Smoking Cessation

—smoking is risky—was quite concise. Repeating the same broad message annually will not attract as much attention as reports touting new aspects of smoking's implications.

The danger is that garnering headlines and television news coverage is not tantamount to public education. In effect, the information is received as fragments on a piecemeal basis rather than through a more comprehensive risk-communication system, which would be better suited to achieving an informed citizenry. An imbalance in resulting risk perceptions can result due to the constraints imposed by using the media as the mechanism for risk communication. The research indicating that perceptions of highly publicized risks are generally not well understood and are usually overestimated should serve as a signal of the limitations of this form of risk communication.

Another source of government information is the warning placed on cigarette packages. These warnings attempt to formalize the state of our scientific knowledge regarding smoking hazards in a succinct way.

Table 2–4 summarizes the evolution of these warnings, which began to be required on cigarette packages and in cigarette advertising in 1965. The action by Congress to mandate warnings was not driven solely by the 1964 smoking report and a perceived need to convey this information to consumers. A variety of states were considering mandatory warnings efforts. For a mass-produced consumer product, the prospect of conflicting state regulations and compliance with a multiplicity of warnings requirements will impose inordinately large costs. A common federal requirement consequently may reduce the warnings costs to firms as well. These considerations led the cigarette industry to support a common labeling requirement.

The initial 1965 warning indicated the probabilistic character of the risks by observing that "Cigarette Smoking May Be Hazardous to Your Health." In 1969 there was less emphasis on the probabilistic aspect, as the warning now declared that "Cigarette Smoking Is Dangerous to Your Health." In addition, the warning began with the human hazard signal word "Warning" rather than "Caution." In the hierarchy of the conventional warnings vocabulary of the American National Standards Institute, "Warning" represents a stronger alert to a potential hazard. In 1984 Congress mandated a series of rotating warnings covering a variety of risks ranging from lung cancer to birth defects.

As the scientific evidence regarding the potential hazards of smoking has become refined, the specificity of the smoking warning increased. Warnings initially alerted potential smokers to the fact that cigarettes were generally "hazardous," but now they detail a variety of particular risks such as cancer and birth defects.

Indication of particular hazards may be of consequence if there is substantial

Table 2–4 Cigarette warning content summaries

Warning period	Warning content[a]
Cigarette warning, 1965	"Caution: Cigarette Smoking May Be Hazardous to Your Health."
Cigarette warning, 1969	"Warning: The Surgeon General Has Determined That Cigarette Smoking Is Dangerous to Your Health."
Cigarette warning, 1984	1. "SURGEON GENERAL'S WARNING: Smoking Causes Lung Cancer, Heart Disease, Emphysema, and May Complicate Pregnancy."
	2. "SURGEON GENERAL'S WARNING: Quitting Smoking Now Greatly Reduces Serious Risks to Your Health."
	3. "SURGEON GENERAL'S WARNING: Smoking by Pregnant Women May Result in Fetal Injury, Premature Birth, and Low Birth Weight."
	4. "SURGEON GENERAL'S WARNING: Cigarette Smoke Contains Carbon Monoxide."

[a]All warnings wording is specified by legislation. See 15 U.S.C. §§ 1331–1341 (1982).

heterogeneity in this risk. If a pregnant woman and, more specifically, the fetus are at substantial risk, a specific warning highlighting this risk may be useful.

Warning about multiple risks also may indicate the specific health risks in more concrete terms and thus may influence the credibility and pertinence of the information. The Federal Trade Commission (FTC) also hypothesized that a series of rotating warnings would foster risk perceptions by providing a fresh message that consumers would be more likely to read.[19] The desirability of rotating warnings is not clear-cut. If some warning messages are more important than others, rotation dilutes the message by presenting it $1/n$ times, where n is the number of warnings being rotated (n currently equals 4). Whether these efforts to bolster the impact of warnings are necessarily desirable depends on how adequately the earlier warnings communicated the risk. The policy objective is informed choice. If elaborations on the structure and content of the warning do not foster more accurate risk perceptions, then they should not be adopted even though they may generate a greater impact.

Although the FTC did review much of the pertinent literature before Congress embarked on the warnings rotation policy, there was no field test of the warnings or determination that the risk probabilities assessed by smokers were inadequate. The failure to undertake such an assessment arose not so much because the government was remiss but because the scientific literature on hazard warnings was not yet well developed. Instead, there was substantial reliance on drawing analogies to product advertising, where firms occasionally rotate their ads to provide a fresh message.

Ascertaining the incremental effect of the different eras of warnings on smoking behavior has proven difficult since the warnings tend to reflect information similar to that being disseminated in the media, particularly through the reports of the Surgeon General. Indeed, studies of cigarette smoking trends have had difficulty in distinguishing any significant independent effect of warnings on smoking behavior.[20] Statistical problems with estimating these impacts do not imply that there has been no downward shift in smoking behavior as a result of risk information. Rather, we simply cannot easily distinguish the incremental effect of the warnings from the effect of information dissemination and changes in the social acceptability of smoking. What we do know with some confidence is that there has been a rise in smoking risk perceptions and a decline in smoking behavior over time, and that there is a linkage between the two.

To put the content of the hazard warnings in perspective, I undertook a field experiment in which respondents from the Chicago area would rate the relative severity of different hazard warnings. This study was undertaken using a group of ninety-nine adult Illinois respondents. The particular warning that I selected to use as a reference point was a variant of the food cancer risk warning adopted under California Proposition 65:

WARNING: This product contains a chemical known to the state of Illinois to cause cancer.

The purpose of the warning was to alert the participants to a potential cancer risk of a product. A separate question in my survey ascertained the total number of cancer deaths to the Illinois population of 11 million from daily consumption of the product. The responses indicated that individuals viewed the risk implied by this warning as being 0.12.[21]

Using this chemical cancer risk warning as the reference point, the survey participants were then asked to indicate whether various warnings implied that the product was less risky than this reference warning, more risky than this reference warning, or as risky as this reference warning. The three warnings that were tested in relationship to the reference risk warning were the 1965 and 1969 cigarette warnings and the warning for saccharin products.

The first warning listed in Table 2–5 is the original 1965 cigarette warning. The second warning appearing in Table 2–5 is a variant of the 1969 cigarette warning, with a statement by the Surgeon General being replaced by the state of Illinois so as to test the overall structure of the warning rather than the cigarette warning per se. The third warning appearing in Table 2–5 is the warning provided for saccharin products. After scientific studies in the 1970s indicated that saccharin posed a potential cancer risk for laboratory animals, particularly in a Canadian study of rats, Congress required that this specific wording be used for saccharin products. The risk level that scientists have assessed for saccharin is a lifetime cancer risk of 40/100,000, or 1/2,500.[22] This risk is consequently of a lower order of magnitude than has been assessed for cigarettes.

Consider first the results for the 1965 cigarette warning. The great majority of the respondents—69 percent of the sample—view this warning as being equivalent to the reference warning indicating that the product causes cancer. The remainder of the respondents are roughly equally divided between believing the product is more or less risky than this reference warning. Recall that the reference warning implied a lifetime cancer risk of .12. As will be detailed in Chapter

Table 2–5 Comparison of the known-to-cause-cancer warning with other wordings

	Compared with the food cancer warning		
Hazard warning	Fraction who regard as less risky	Fraction who regard as equally risky	Fraction who regard as more risky
1965 cigarette warning 1. Caution: Use of this product may be hazardous to your health.	.14	.69	.17
Variant of 1969 cigarette warning 2. Warning: The state of Illinois has determined that this product is dangerous to your health.	.36	.48	.16
Saccharin warning 3. Use of this product may be hazardous to your health. This product contains a chemical that has been determined to cause cancer in laboratory animals.	.56	.18	.26

Source: Viscusi (1988), p. 307.

4, the incremental lifetime death risk from lung cancer to a smoker is on the order of .05 to .10, and the total smoking mortality rate is on the order of .18 to .36, based on 1991 studies.[23] Scientific estimates of the magnitude of the risk in 1965—the time of the warning—were closer to the assessed risk levels. Pinpoint optimality in a risk communication is an unreasonable standard. Overall, this warning appears to be generally consistent with the estimated smoking risk level.

Furthermore, the warning alone is not the sole source of information provided. It is but one component of the risk information that individuals utilize in forming their risk perceptions. Nevertheless, this comparison of the risk equivalent implied by the warning is an instructive measure of the extent to which the warnings policy is fostering accurate risk perceptions.

Although there was no evidence in the 1960s to indicate that the 1965 warning was inadequate, Congress altered the content of the warning in an effort to strengthen the warning's message. The second warning in Table 2–5 is a modified version of the 1969 cigarette warning used within the context of a food safety survey. An almost identical fraction of the respondents view the product as being more risky than the reference warning, but there has been a shift of about one-fifth of the respondents who formerly viewed the product as being equally risky to the reference warning and who now view the product as being less risky. Somewhat surprisingly, this warning seems to suggest that the wording of the 1969 warning conveyed less risk than did the 1965 warning. This result may stem in part from respondents' belief that the first warning in Table 2–5, which is an unaltered version of the 1965 warning, was more directly related to cigarettes than was the warning that modified the 1969 cigarette warning. The second warning in Table 2.5 omits the specific reference to the Surgeon General included in the 1969 cigarette warning. Nevertheless, these results do suggest that the change in warning language did not greatly affect the public perception of the risk. Indeed, this warning may not have led to any improvement in the accuracy of the risks being communicated.

The final reference point is the warning for saccharin. As one would expect, this warning indicates a potential cancer risk for laboratory animals that poses a lower risk than do the other two cigarette warnings. Over half of the sample view the saccharin warning as implying less risk than the reference warning. At the other extreme, more people believe the saccharin warning implies a higher risk than does the reference warning. This wide divergence of opinion suggests that it is very difficult for people to extrapolate from evidence regarding laboratory animal tests. There is the potential for extreme responses in both directions. In contrast, the implications of the cigarette warnings are more tightly clustered. The variance in responses to the first and second warnings in Table 2–5—the two variants of the cigarette warning—is much less. These warnings are tantamount to simply indicating to consumers that the product causes cancer.

Media Coverage

Government dissemination of information is not the only source of public information available to smokers. Nor did the mid-1960s mark the advent of the public provision of information about smoking risks. The hazards of smoking have long been covered by the media, and they have received substantial attention over a number of decades.

One instructive measure of the continuity of the media coverage is the tally of articles dealing with smoking hazards that have appeared in *Reader's Digest*, which appears in Table 2–6. This magazine provides a mix of articles from a variety of publications. The selection of articles is not a random sample of articles published. Indeed, the publication has a long history of publishing a large number of antismoking articles and not accepting cigarette advertising.[24] However, even though this publication has an antismoking orientation, this editorial policy would not distort the main matter of interest—the trend in number of articles, not the actual article count. The percentage of antismoking articles will simply be higher than for other publications, such as *Newsweek* and *U.S. News & World Report*. There would have to be a shift in the editorial policy with respect to the relative emphasis on cigarette articles for the article trends not to be a meaningful index of changes in media attention.

The frequency of articles addressing smoking hazards is somewhat intermittent. There is evidence of spurts in media attention for smoking issues, as in the case of other media topics. In 1984, for example, there were five articles dealing with cigarette smoking, and in 1976, there was a record number of six smoking articles.[25]

In terms of the broad trends, there is evidence of consistent coverage of smoking risks in *Reader's Digest*, but there is some upward trend to this coverage, as is clearer from the article counts by decade in the bottom panel of Table 2–6. In the 1950s there were a total of twelve articles dealing with smoking risks, a result that is noteworthy since it antedates the 1964 smoking report and the 1965 imposition of cigarette warnings. By the 1960s the smoking risk article total per decade had risen to seventeen, and there has been a slight increase in the number of articles in the subsequent two decades.

Smoking does not represent an issue that emerged only recently. Rather, these risks have received consistent but increasing media attention over a three-decade period. Although the degree of confidence that we have in the scientific information pertaining to the effects of smoking has increased over time, it is clear that there has long been available a substantial set of information that would enable the public to form a belief that there are potential risks of smoking. It would be surprising given this extensive and increasing coverage if there were no public awareness of smoking hazards.

CIGARETTE ADVERTISING

Another source of information for potential smokers is that provided by cigarette advertising. Cigarettes have long been among the most highly advertised consumer products, with an annual advertising budget now in excess of $1 billion and a promotional budget greater than $2 billion annually.[26] In some years there have been more ads for cigarettes than for any other consumer product.[27]

Table 2–6 Number of articles relating to smoking and health risks in *Reader's Digest,* 1950–1988

	Year	No. of articles
Annual article counts	1989	2
	1988	3
	1987	2
	1986	2
	1985	4
	1984	5
	1983	1
	1982	2
	1981	1
	1980	1
	1979	0
	1978	1
	1977	0
	1976	6
	1975	2
	1974	0
	1973	3
	1972	3
	1971	2
	1970	2
	1969	1
	1968	2
	1967	1
	1966	2
	1965	2
	1964	3
	1963	3
	1962	3
	1961	0
	1960	0
	1959	2
	1958	3
	1957	2
	1956	2
	1955	0
	1954	2
	1953	1
	1950–1952	0
	Total:	71
Article counts by decade	1950–1959	12
	1960–1969	17
	1970–1979	19
	1980–1989	23

Advertising is not always tantamount to product advocacy. Particularly for mature products such as cigarettes, the main purpose of advertising is to encourage brand switching rather than to draw new customers into the market. As a result, firms often engage in competitive advertising, including claims that their brand has less of a negative product attribute than others. Recent automobile ads, for example, indicate that one line of cars is less risky than competitors' cars. Similar types of comparison-style risk information have been included in cigarette ads for the past several decades. In recent years cigarette ads have included the mandatory warning of the Surgeon General as part of the ad. However, even before the inclusion of this information, cigarette advertising frequently included reference to the health aspects of cigarettes.

Because of the prominence of consumer concerns regarding the health consequences of smoking, one potential way for a cigarette manufacturer to gain a competitive advantage is to make claims that its product is comparatively less harmful in that regard. Making health claims of this type should increase the prominence of health concerns among potential smokers, thus decreasing the overall market for cigarettes. For those who are reassured by such ads, the opposite result will be true. From the standpoint of the firm making the claims, the comparative advertising is potentially beneficial to the extent that it shifts smokers from other brands to its brand.

Figure 2–4 illustrates the character of the health information with three cigarette advertisements. The 1935 Camel ad suggests that a Camel smoker is less likely to become winded since it is a "milder" cigarette. The 1953 Kent ad, which is typical of filter cigarette ads, touts the ability of cigarette filters to remove tar and other controversial compounds from cigarette smoke.[28] The 1971 L&M ad in Figure 2–4 reflects the quantitative approach to health risk exposures that has become typical of the ads used for low-tar cigarettes.

The character and form of the information vary, but what is most noteworthy is that a negative attribute of the product (for example, tar) plays a prominent role in the ad. Although an ad might suggest that a product has a lower value of tar, the mere mention of this negative attribute is highly unusual since it draws consumers' attention to an undesirable feature of cigarettes.

In his influential book *Unsafe at Any Speed*, Ralph Nader (1972) observed that efforts by the Ford Motor Company to sell cars on the basis of their safety in the early 1950s did not succeed since it called consumers' attention to a negative attribute, product risk. The message from the market was simple: Safety does not sell. In 1953 *Business Week* questioned the economic wisdom of the industry's advertising strategy: "Why has the industry persisted in this negative form of advertising even when, as tobacco growers and others complain, it hurts the trade by making people conscious that cigarettes may be harmful?"[29]

Advertising the comparatively lower risk of a brand name may hurt that brand if individuals pay excessive attention to the presence of a risk rather than its lower level. Moreover, it may stigmatize the entire product group. Although safety appears to have become more marketable in the postregulatory era of the 1980s and 1990s (see, for example, the Volvo automobile ads from that period), the advertising environment of the previous decades in which these ads appeared

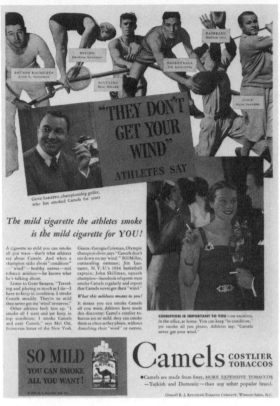

Figure 2—4A Camel ad, 1935

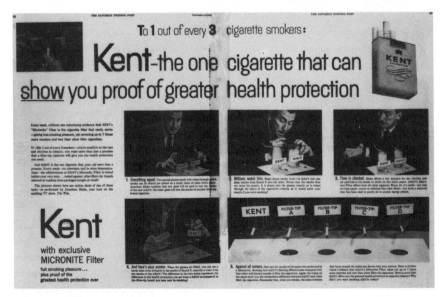

Figure 2—4B Kent ad, 1953

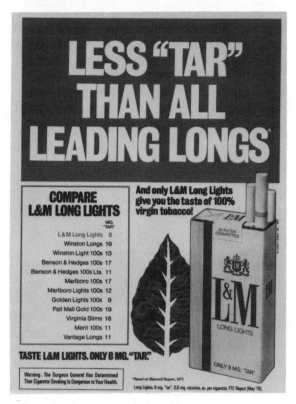

Figure 2–4C   L&M ad, 1979

was quite different. The willingness to mention health risks in an ad is an implicit recognition that the safety of the product was a salient consumer concern.

Advertising with respect to the health consequences of smoking has taken a variety of forms. Most recently, firms have touted the low tar and nicotine contents of their cigarettes. In earlier years the presence of a filter for the cigarette was highlighted as a potentially beneficial health-related attribute. Even before the claims regarding these two aspects of cigarettes became prominent, there were competitive advertising claims regarding the comparative safety of different brands of cigarettes.

Indeed, the period from 1957 to 1960 marked an advertising war among the cigarette companies, which highlighted the lowest tar and nicotine levels of particular cigarette brands. The low-tar ads quickly proliferated.[30] Kent improved its filter and declared "significantly less tar and nicotine than any other filter brand." Other companies followed suit: "Today's Marlboro—22% less tar, 34% less nicotine," and "lowest tar of all lo-tar cigarettes" (Duke cigarettes).

During this three-year period known as the great "tar derby," market competition led to accurate tar and nicotine information being provided to consumers, who responded by purchasing cigarettes with an average of one-third less tar and nicotine than before.[31] This advertising was stymied by a 1960 industrywide agreement to eliminate this tar and nicotine advertising, which had been brought about by the FTC. Through this action the government initially played an obstructionist role in the dissemination of tar and nicotine information.[32] Although the exact reason for the FTC policy remains unclear, even to FTC officials, one prominent factor is that the U.S. Surgeon General had made recommendations against smoking low-tar cigarettes.[33] The Surgeon General had adopted a purist anticigarette industry stance rather than making a more refined distinction that would foster market competition to promote safety. This position was not shared by all health groups. The American Cancer Society recognized the ill-conceived nature of discouraging tar and nicotine advertising and urged the FTC to reverse its policy and let the cigarette companies resume their tar derby. In the late 1960s the FTC reversed its position and encouraged advertising of tar and nicotine content. In 1967 the FTC published tar and nicotine levels for cigarettes, and in 1971 all cigarette advertising was required to include tar and nicotine levels as a result of a voluntary cigarette manufacturers' agreement.

The most extensive study of long-term trends in cigarette advertising is that of Ringold and Calfee (1989), who examined advertising trends from 1926 to 1986 for seven major brands. These included brands that were among the leading sellers several decades ago, such as Camel, Chesterfield, and Old Gold. Moreover, it also included the best-selling filter cigarette and largest-selling cigarette overall—Marlboro.

Table 2–7 summarizes the aspects of the ads that were in Ringold and Calfee's sample. The content of advertising spans a variety of attributes of cigarettes, including their construction, taste, and price. The most important concern from the standpoint of our examination of advertising is the degree to which health claims were prominent. Overall, 14.9 percent of the claims made with respect to cigarettes were the mandatory health claims, and 12.2 percent were voluntary health-related claims. The combined share of the mandatory and voluntary health claims constituted over one-fourth of all the claims made with respect to cigarettes. The leading cigarette in terms of health claims is Kent, for which 40.5 percent of all of the claims made were health-related. The Kent ad in Figure 2–4 exemplifies the type of approach used for these cigarettes. Kent cigarettes were the first popular filter brand of cigarettes, so the prominence of health concerns is not unexpected given the nature of this product.

Table 2–8 provides a more detailed breakdown of the character of the health-related claims as well as the time period in which they were made. Even as early as the 1920s, health claims were a prominent part of cigarette advertising. Although the sample included only seventeen health-related claims over the 1926–1929 period, the number of ads reflected in this sample is not that great, so the relative share of health claims is fairly large. In particular, 18 percent of all cigarette claims made in advertising were health-related during that time period. The most prominent form of advertising pertained to claims that a particular brand was less harmful than other brands with respect to the major adverse effects that have been linked to smoking: effects on the throat, coughs, lungs, mouth, and lips. These claims were generally of a comparative nature, in which

Table 2–7 Claims by brand: Longitudinal set (category as a percent of total claims within brand)

	Camel	Chesterfield	Old Gold	Viceroy	Lucky Strike	Marlboro	Kent	Total
Number of ads	61	48	44	46	56	59	34	348
Number of claims	456	291	270	320	310	307	232	2186
Claims per ad	7.5	6.1	6.1	7.0	5.5	5.2	6.8	6.3
Claims by type								
Cigarette construction	14.0%	23.7%	24.1%	21.9%	26.5%	24.1%	19.4%	21.5%
Taste	20.8	27.1	18.9	14.7	17.7	14.7	15.9	18.7
Exhortation to buy/slogan	11.8	11.0	8.5	8.4	16.5	17.3	6.5	11.7
Competitive advantage	9.4	7.2	8.5	5.9	6.5	5.2	8.6	7.4
Mandatory health	13.4	3.8	11.9	16.3	13.9	20.5	27.6	14.9
Voluntary health	14.5	4.1	13.3	20.3	11.6	6.8	12.9	12.2
Health (combined)	27.9	7.9	25.2	36.6	25.5	27.3	40.5	27.1
Utility[a]	8.3	15.8	7.8	4.7	2.6	2.9	7.3	7.0
Availability	0.7	0.7	1.1	0.9	0.3	0.7	—	0.6
Endorsements	4.4	2.4	0.4	0.9	2.9	—	0.4	1.9
Premium/contest	0.4	1.4	3.7	0.6	0.3	1.0	—	1.0
Price	1.8	2.1	1.1	3.1	—	6.5	1.3	2.3
War bonds/union made	0.4	0.7	0.7	2.2	1.3	0.3	—	0.8
Total	100%	100%	100%	100%	100%	100%	100%	100%

Source: Ringold and Calfee (1989).

[a] Utility includes pleasure, satisfaction, and self-reward.

the better performance of the particular cigarette being advertised was emphasized.

Very few of the health claims suggested that overall cigarettes were beneficial to one's health. Positive health claims, including testimonials by doctors and athletes, were usually more specific. In some cases the ads claim that cigarettes aided digestion, provided relaxation, improved one's concentration, or improved one's disposition. However, because of the emergence of adverse health-risk information, the impact of the advertising was at least partly negative when processed by viewers of the ad.

Also striking is the extent to which advertising became a vehicle for communicating findings in the scientific and medical literature. Almost one-fifth of all the health claims pertain to the citation of scientific and medical research. These citations are in addition to the mandatory references to the warning by the Surgeon General that are reflected in the advertising data periods beginning in 1970. Even ads that do not cite specific studies, such as the L&M ad in Figure 2–4, are more technical in nature than the typical product advertising.

Table 2–8 Health claims by period: Longitudinal set (category as a percent of total health claims within period)

					Years				
	1926–1929	1930–1939	1940–1949	1950–1954	1955–1959	1960–1969	1970–1979	1980–1986	Total
Number of health claims	17	69	62	65	12	9	223	135	592
Claim types									
Throat	23.5%	21.7%	17.7%	16.9%	8.3%	11.1%	—	—	7.3
Coughs	17.6	13.0	—	—	—	—	—	—	2.0
Lungs	—	—	—	4.6	—	—	—	—	0.5
Mouth	—	4.3	4.8	7.7	—	—	—	—	1.9
Lips	—	14.5	8.1	—	8.3	—	—	—	2.4
Unspecified irritation	11.8	4.3	4.8	4.6	8.3	22.2	—	—	2.0
Reduce worry about smoking	5.9	4.3	1.6	4.6	16.7	—	—	—	2.0
Health protection	11.8	8.7	1.6	12.3	—	—	—	—	2.9
Teeth	—	1.4	11.3	1.5	—	—	—	—	1.5
Taste buds	5.9	1.4	—	1.5	—	11.1	—	—	0.7
Colds/flu	—	—	—	1.5	—	—	—	—	0.2

Aids digestion	—	2.9	—	—	—	—	—	—	0.3
Relaxer	11.8	7.2	1.6	1.5	8.3	11.1	—	—	1.9
Improves concentration	—	5.8	1.6	—	—	—	—	—	0.7
Improves disposition	—	1.4	—	—	16.7	—	—	—	0.7
Fitness	5.9	4.3	—	—	—	—	—	—	0.7
Habit	—	—	—	1.5	—	—	—	—	0.2
Citation of scientific research	—	4.3	11.3	12.3	—	22.2	23.3	22.2	17.2
Citation of medical research	5.9	—	1.6	3.1	—	—	—	—	0.7
Medical/dental endorsement	—	—	11.3	4.6	—	—	—	—	1.7
Nicotine figures	—	—	1.6	—	—	—	23.3	23.0	14.0
Reduced nicotine	—	—	12.9	13.8	16.7	—	1.3	—	3.7
Tar figures	—	—	—	—	—	—	23.3	23.0	13.9
Reduced tar	—	—	8.1	7.7	16.7	—	6.7	10.4	6.9
Surgeon General's warning	—	—	—	—	—	—	22.0	23.0	13.5
Total	100%	100%	100%	100%	100%	100%	100%	100%	100%

Source: Ringold and Calfee (1989).

CONCLUSION

There are several models one could use to analyze smoking behavior—the rational economic choice model, a cognitive processes model, or a framework that suggests that smoking is the result of irrational or random decisions. Except perhaps in the final instance, the information that individuals have about the risk will play a fundamental role. In the case of the fully rational model, the provision of risk information will induce accurate risk perceptions and informed choices. In the case of the model of choice with cognitive limitations, additional information may improve or worsen the choice, depending on the character of the risk information. For example, the risks of highly publicized events tend to be overestimated. Similarly, individuals tend to overestimate the small risks that they face and underestimate the larger hazards that they may encounter. The role of these influences is unclear since smoking risks are highly publicized but also tend to be fairly large. As a result, there are competing biases that will influence the overall net direction of bias in smoking risk perceptions.

Individuals are not born with these risk perceptions. Rather, these beliefs are influenced by the various types of information they receive about smoking and acquire through their smoking experiences. A review of the private and social forms of information provision suggests that these efforts have a long history and have been quite extensive.

The main implication of the results pertaining to smoking risk information is that the public concern with the health consequences of smoking did not begin with the on-product labels of cigarettes or with the official publications by the Surgeon General. These concerns were prominent in the media and were reflected in the advertising for cigarettes. This information also will influence risk perceptions people have with respect to cigarettes. The character of these risk perceptions as they have evolved through the past half century will be the subject of the following chapter.

NOTES

1. U.S. Department of Health and Human Services (1989), pp. 22, 160. The other deaths include those due to smoking-related fires, birth defects, and secondhand smoke.

2. U.S. Department of Health, Education, and Welfare, (1964).

3. U.S. Department of Health and Human Services (1988).

4. See U.S. Department of Health and Human Services (1989), p. 88, for documentation of the decline.

5. Schelling (1984) and Schwartz (1989) provide an economic discussion of the "addiction" issue. The psychologists' perspective on addiction is reflected in Eiser (1983) and in Eiser and VanDer Pligt (1986).

6. Suppose that smoking poses either a high risk H or a low risk L and that the consumer has received a single piece of risk information—a hazard warning. Then the assessed probability P that this is a high-risk activity is given by

$$P(H|\text{warning}) = \frac{P(\text{warning}|H)\ P(H)}{P(\text{warning}|H)\ P(H)\ +\ P(\text{warning}|L)\ P(L)}.$$

7. See Fischhoff et al. (1981).

8. See Viscusi (1985a,b).

9. For discussion of this phenomenon using data from the United Kingdom, see Marsh (1985).

10. See Kahneman and Tversky (1979).

11. See the discussions in Combs and Slovic (1979); Fischhoff et al. (1981); Lichtenstein et al. (1978); Slovic, Fischhoff, and Lichtenstein (1979); Viscusi (1985a,b, 1988); Viscusi and Magat (1987); Viscusi, Magat, and Huber (1987); and Wildavsky (1988).

12. See Viscusi (1985a,b).

13. The four groups of respondents participating in this study included forty members of the League of Women Voters, thirty college students, twenty-five business and professional people who are members of what is known as the "active club" in Eugene, Oregon, and a group of fifteen "experts." These experts included individuals with some professional background in the risk area, such as geographers, economists, a lawyer, and a biologist. It should be emphasized that this expert-opinion group does not serve as the objective reference point in the same way as do the government studies of cigarette smoking risks that will be used as the reference point in Chapter 3. They do, however, provide an interesting contrast between the opinions of average citizens and the opinions of more informed citizens.

14. In particular, workers revised their probabilistic beliefs in the correct direction and in a manner that was consistent with Bayesian learning.

15. Similarly, the subsequent study of hazard warnings for radon risk exposures by Smith et al. (1988,1990) indicate that there is both understanding of the risk information communicated as well as learning in the correct direction. Once again, however, these studies do not imply fully accurate perceptions, only behavior that is broadly consistent with a rational learning process.

16. See Viscusi (1988).

17. U.S. Department of Health, Education, and Welfare (1964).

18. The Surgeon General is required to issue this annual report under the Public Health Cigarette Smoking Act of 1969.

19. U.S. Federal Trade Commission (1981). There was, however, no scientific evidence to support the hypothesis. The warnings-rotation experience in Sweden, for example, was instituted along with other smoking policy changes.

20. A good discussion of this and related issues appears in Calfee (1985), and Schneider, Klein, and Murphy (1981).

21. The overall cancer death risk indicated by the warning dwarfs the 1/100,000 lifetime cancer risk threshold for which the warning was designed. Fortunately, this warnings policy has never been fully implemented, so that the full effects of this unduly alarmist policy have never been fully manifested.

22. See Travis et al. (1987) at p. 417.

23. See Chapter 4 for a detailed derivation. The risk range is based on 1991 studies.

24. U.S. Department of Health and Human Services (1989), p. 508.

25. The focus of these articles has changed somewhat over time, as the 1976 articles dealt primarily with different hazards of smoking, whereas in 1984 three of the articles addressed strategies for stopping smoking while two focused on smoking risks.

26. *Morbidity and Mortality Weekly Report*, 39 no. 16 (April 27, 1990), p. 263.

27. See the U.S. Federal Trade Commission (1981), pp. 2–3, and more generally, Warner (1986).

28. The Kent micronite filter has become an object of legal controversy, since it included asbestos, which is now known to be a highly potent carcinogen. The courts have

yet to rule on whether any cases of mesothelioma (a form of cancer that is a signature disease linked almost exclusively to asbestos) among former smokers can be traced to their smoking behavior.

29. "Cigarette Scare: What'll the Trade Do?" *Business Week*, December 5, 1953, p. 60.
30. The text of these ads is from Calfee (1986), p. 36.
31. See Calfee (1985). The averaging is on a sales-weighted basis.
32. See Calfee (1985), p. 5.
33. See Calfee (1985), p. 45.

3
Long-Term Trends in
Attitudes toward Smoking

The substantial provision of smoking risk information should lead rational consumers to form reasonable perceptions of the risk. The stylized consumer profiled in Chapter 2 will ignore this information, whereas the risk perceptions of consumers with cognitive limitations may err in either direction, depending on which type of bias is of greatest consequence. This chapter will explore the validity of these alternative views by assessing the character of smoking risk perceptions. Do individuals understand the hazards posed by smoking? What have been the trends in these risk perceptions? How have smoking rates changed as risk perceptions have increased? In the next chapters we will refine this assessment using more detailed data from particular time periods, primarily 1985, whereas here it affords us a long-term perspective on smoking risks.

The smoking debate reached substantial prominence in the 1980s and 1990s, but it began much earlier. Moreover, even though most of the major smoking policies have been instituted within the last twenty-five years, the policy issues pertaining to smoking risk perceptions are not new. As early as 1642, Pope Urban VIII threatened to excommunicate those who smoked tobacco.[1] Public debate over the hazards of smoking and the consideration of policy actions to address smoking risks began to most closely resemble the current situation following the introduction of the mass marketing of cigarettes. James Buchanan Duke[2] introduced mechanization into the cigarette industry in 1884, and by 1889 he was marketing 1 billion cigarettes per year.[3] This widespread utilization of cigarettes led to selected policy initiatives not unlike many policies considered in recent years:

> Beginning with Washington in 1893, no fewer than 14 states outlawed the sale, manufacture, possession, advertising and/or use of cigarettes, aka coffin nails, little white slavers, dope sticks, paper pills, brain capsules, coffin pills, and devil's kindling wood. At least 21 other states and territories considered cigarette prohibition.
>
> Congress was asked to protect the public health by requiring that cigarette packages be stamped with a skull and crossbones, and labelled "POISON." Many employers refused to hire cigarette smokers. Non-smokers said their health was being jeopardized by "secondhand smoke."[4]

In this chapter I will be concerned with the evolution and level of these risk perceptions, focusing primarily on the recent era. The main source of information for tracking the evolution of smoking perceptions is public opinion polls of assessments of smoking hazards. These polls provide time trends in public perceptions of smoking risks and the public's willingness to impose restrictions on smoking behavior. Antismoking attitudes of various kinds have long been prevalent, but recently there has been increased prominence of smoking issues, particularly with respect to society's willingness to take policy actions. What is perhaps most striking is that the increased provision of smoking risk information has been mirrored in the shifts in public perceptions of smoking.

PUBLIC OPINION SURVEY DATA ON SMOKING

The most continuous series of public opinion poll data is the Gallup Poll results, which have tracked awareness of smoking risks from 1949 to the present. Relying on these data is not ideal. The wording of the questions pertaining to the risk does not elicit a specific probability judgment regarding the hazards of smoking. Rather, the questions are typically more vaguely worded. The survey questions ascertain whether respondents believe that cigarette smoking is "harmful." However, the risk threshold as to what constitutes harm may differ across individuals so that the implications of designating any particular risk as harmful are not necessarily uniform across respondents. In addition, even for any particular respondent we do not know what it means for a product to be "harmful." Does this mean that the product causes certain injury, that the risk of injury is above one chance in ten, that the risk is more severe than for other products? Other surveys involving qualitative risk questions are similarly flawed. A 1980 Roper Poll concluded that 31 percent of smokers did not know that smoking "greatly" increased their risk of heart attack.[5] How large a risk increase must be for it to be "great" is unclear.

An additional problem is that the subjective risk cutoffs for labeling an activity risky vary across individuals. My study of perceptions of job risks for workers on blue-collar jobs in the chemical industry indicates the types of problems that can arise.[6] Workers rated their jobs on a quantitative scale in terms of the annual frequency of an on-the-job injury. They also answered a qualitative question pertaining to whether their job exposed them to dangerous or unhealthy conditions. The absolute risk cutoff that workers could tolerate before they labeled their jobs "dangerous" varied substantially with educational background. College-educated workers had a danger threshold of an annual injury frequency rate of .06, whereas workers who did not go to college had a danger cutoff of .09. Less-educated workers were able to accept a higher risk before designating the job dangerous. Across-person comparisons of qualitative risk variables consequently may be invalid, but comparison over time for relatively stable population groups should be more reliable.

As a result, analyzing the opinion poll questions can provide information on trends in risk awareness but cannot resolve the issue of whether the absolute level of risk perceptions is sufficient. Perceptions may be biased in either direction irrespective of a perception that smoking is "harmful." The main focus of this book consequently will be on the risk questions considered in Chapter 4, which are based on a meaningful, well-defined probabilistic metric.

Notwithstanding these shortcomings, the survey data provide a mechanism for tracking the development of risk perceptions over time and for establishing the comparability of risk perceptions for lung cancer with the risk perceptions for other classes of hazards posed by cigarettes. These results consequently will be suggestive in indicating the likely generalizability of the lung cancer results considered in subsequent chapters. Moreover, the cigarette warnings mandated by Congress are also qualitative in nature so that it is useful to obtain a sense of the degree to which respondents believe in other qualitative statements of the risk.

To establish a comparable measure of shifts in risk perceptions, it is necessary to track questions pertaining to particular classes of risks over time. Table 3–1 summarizes these survey results for lung cancer and throat cancer. Inspection of the vertical columns in Table 3–1 enables one to track the evolution of the responses of particular population segments to this class of hazards. In 1954 the survey asked whether cigarette smoking was "one of the causes of lung cancer." In 1957 there was a minor modification of the question, which then asked whether it was "one of the causes of cancer of the lung." This wording change should have had little impact on the nature of the responses. Similarly, the wording used in 1971 and thereafter, which is whether the respondent thinks that cigarette smoking "is/not one of the causes of lung cancer," should yield almost identical results, as in fact appears to be the case. Comparison of the findings for 1969 and 1971 indicates no shift in responses accompanying the change in phrasing.

Table 3–1 Gallup Poll opinion surveys, 1949–1981: Questions on cigarette smoking and cancer (% responding positively)

Question	Year	All respondents	Cigarette smokers	Non–cigarette smokers	Former cigarette smokers
Cigarette smoking one of causes of lung cancer?	1954	41	30	48	54
One of causes of cancer of lung?	7/1957	50	38	59	—
	12/1957	47	35	—	—
	1958	44	33	—	—
	1958[a]	45	33	—	—
	1969	70	—	—	—
Is/is not one cause of lung cancer?	1971[b]	71	—	—	—
	1972	70	—	—	—
	1977	81	72	87	—
	1981	83	69	91	—
Smoking as cause of throat cancer?	1977	79	73	82	—
	1981	81	69	87	—

[a]Special survey.

[b]Survey taken in nine different nations, but this figure is for U.S. responses only.

The responses of cigarette smokers and nonsmokers to the lung cancer questions follow the same relative pattern. Since the population group breakdowns are not available for all years, consider first the answers by the entire population. The assessment of lung cancer risks appears to have moved in discontinuous increments. In the 1950s, 40 to 50 percent of the population expressed awareness of lung cancer risks. By the 1970s, this figure had jumped to 70 percent, and by the 1980s over 80 percent of the population believed that cigarette smoking was a cause of lung cancer.

As one might expect, 5 to 10 percent more nonsmokers were likely to regard smoking as posing a lung cancer risk. Since individuals who believe that smoking is harmful should be less likely to pursue this activity if they are behaving in a rational manner, the higher risk awareness for nonsmokers is consistent with such a selection process.

The throat cancer questions have been less regular but appear to track the pattern of lung cancer risk questions very closely. Thus, roughly the same percentage of respondents who view cigarette smoking to be a cause of lung cancer also view smoking to be a cause of throat cancer.

Other patterns of risk perception are similar in their general character. Smoking risk perceptions were even widespread over four decades ago. As the figures in Table 3–2 indicate, in 1949 over half of all smokers and two-thirds of nonsmokers regarded cigarette smoking as being "harmful." The great majority of the population regarded smoking as a risky pursuit, and although this does not represent a universal perception, it does indicate a substantial awareness of the risks. By 1981, 90 percent of the population viewed smoking as being "harmful," and now this figure is even higher (see Figure 2–3). There has consequently been a substantial rise in risk perceptions. By 1980 it was almost universally believed that cigarette smoking is dangerous in some respect. As in 1949, more nonsmokers than cigarette smokers believe that such hazards are present.

The fact that some small segment of the population does not believe that

Table 3–2 Gallup Poll opinion surveys, 1949–1981: Questions on cigarette smoking and health risks (% responding positively)

Question	Year	All respondents	Cigarette smokers	Non–cigarette smokers
Cigarette smoking harmful?	1949	—	52	66
	1977	90	83	95
	1981	90	80	96
Smoking one cause of heart disease?	7/1957	38	32	43
	1969	60	—	—
	1977	68	63	72
	1981	74	59	82
Smoking one cause of birth defects?	1977	41	30	49
	1981	53	34	64
Relation between smoking and other diseases?	7/1957	38	—	—

smoking is harmful does not mean that they equate not being harmful with being risk-free. One can view each respondent as having some threshold risk value, above which a product is classified as harmful. The fact that cigarettes may not be above this threshold implies only that the respondents believe the risk is not so great that it passes the harmful-risk cutoff. What makes interpretation of the responses even more difficult is that the cutoff may differ across the population. If, however, the mix of risk cutoffs for considering smoking "harmful" is not changing over time, these opinion poll results provide a reasonable index of the change in smokers' risk perceptions.

The pattern of risk perceptions with respect to heart disease shown in Table 3–2 is similar to that for lung cancer except that the level of risk perceptions is somewhat lower. This pattern is what one would expect since the lung cancer risk has long been the best documented and most highly publicized risk of smoking. Whereas 50 percent of the population in 1957 viewed smoking as a cause of lung cancer, only 30 percent of the population had similar views about the cigarette smoking-heart disease linkage. The extent of the change in the heart disease perception has been greater than that for lung cancer, no doubt in part because of the lower initial risk perception in earlier years. Whereas the fraction of the population viewing cigarettes as being a cause of lung cancer rose by 23 percentage points from 1957 to 1981, there was a 36-point increase in the percentage of the population believing that cigarettes are a cause of heart disease.

A much smaller group of individuals—just over half of the population in 1981—viewed smoking to be a cause of birth defects. The birth defect linkage is less generally understood, and the main policy issue that the survey structure does not completely resolve is whether the target population of women of child-bearing age has received the information and has reasonable risk perceptions. Although precise data are not available on risk perceptions for all population segments, 46 percent of all females believe that cigarette smoking is a cause of birth defects as opposed to 36 percent of males, so that there is some evidence of appropriate informational targeting. Evidence from the National Health Interview Survey indicates that by the mid-1980s, three-fourths of all women believed that smoking increases the risks of premature birth (76 percent), still birth (68 percent), miscarriage (75 percent), having a low-birth-weight baby (85 percent), and stroke (if also taking birth control pills, 72 percent).[7]

The final set of results in Table 3–2 pertains to the percentage who believe that there is a relationship between cigarette smoking and unsuspected other diseases (a question that was asked in 1957). This question yielded the same fraction of individuals identifying a risk link as those who also believe that there was a causal cigarette smoking-heart disease relationship.

For the four decades for which we have survey information, the prevalence of a perception of smoking risks has been quite substantial and increasing. Although lung cancer has been the most prominently identified hazard, there is evidence of similarly held risk perceptions for throat cancer. Moreover, the extent of awareness of a linkage between cigarette smoking and heart disease and between cigarette smoking and other disease is now not too far behind.

Evidence of increasingly widespread awareness of smoking risks does not, however, imply that levels of risk perceptions are accurate, only that a growing portion of the population regards smoking to be hazardous in some respect. Ideally, one would want all individuals to have correct perceptions of the risk. Survey trends suggest that there is a broader dissemination of knowledge about the class of risks posed by cigarettes, which is one index of a better-informed citizenry.

Public concern with taking policy actions to decrease smoking in various ways also provides information on the extent of risk perceptions and societal attitudes toward smoking more generally. Table 3–3 summarizes the Gallup Poll responses to a variety of policy options. Informational alternatives such as warnings for cigarettes, antismoking efforts, and antismoking television ads have long had substantial, but by no means universal, support. The most popular of these measures is the distribution of literature to schoolchildren—a policy that was favored by 68 percent of all respondents in 1957. Support for completely banning cigarette advertising has risen over time from 36 percent in 1977 to 55 percent in 1988, which reflects increasingly widespread support for restricting firms' ability to distribute positive forms of information about their product. Restrictions on the sale and use of cigarettes have differing popularity depending on the breadth

Table 3–3 Gallup Poll opinion surveys, 1962–1988: Questions on cigarette policy issues (% responding positively)

				Year			
Question	1957	1962	1977	1978	1981	1987	1988
Smoking danger great enough so health department should warn?	53						
Distribute literature to schoolchildren?	68		51				
Desire law against selling cigarettes to those under age 16?		79					
Law against allowing under age 16 to smoke/no law against same?		56					
Ban cigarette sales completely?			19				
Complete ban on cigarette ads?			36		43	49	55
Smoking on commercial airplanes should/shouldn't be banned completely?				43			
Amount of $ HEW spends on antismoking television/radio ads?				51			
What policy should be followed re: smoking in public places (trains, bus, airplanes, restaurants, offices)?							
No restrictions?			10				
Specified area set for smoker?			68				
No smoking?			16				
Complete ban on smoking in all public places? (flavor)						55	60

of the measures. Whereas 79 percent of the population favored a law banning the sale of cigarettes to children under the age of 16 in 1962, only 19 percent of all respondents in 1977 favored a complete cigarette sale ban.

The questions with the greatest continuity over time that permit us to track the change in attitudes toward smoking policies are those pertaining to restrictions on smoking. These questions are also noteworthy since they represent the most remarkable shift in public perceptions, which far outweighs the change in risk perceptions identified in Tables 3–1 and 3–2.

In 1977, 68 percent of the population favored setting aside specified areas in public places for smokers, and only 16 percent of the population favored a no-smoking requirement. Similarly, in 1978, 43 percent of the population believed that cigarette smoking on commercial airplanes should be banned completely.

By 1988, social acceptability of smoking had plummeted. A surprisingly large 60 percent of the population favored a complete ban on smoking in all public places—not simply airplanes. The most comparable question to this in earlier years is the 16 percent of respondents favoring no-smoking areas in 1977, indicating a surge of support for increasingly stringent smoking restrictions. Advocacy of strong antismoking policy measures has clearly increased, and this shift has been much greater than the prevalence of smoking risk awareness.

The shift in policy views may be due to the increased belief that smoking is hazardous not only to the smoker but to others as well. Moreover, there is a dwindling number of smokers, which has affected the character of the social debate. Smoking has virtually disappeared among the most vocal and articulate segment of society. It has become more acceptable for a large nonsmoking majority to impose restrictions on the shrinking smoking population.

CHANGES IN SMOKING BEHAVIOR

The relationship of the change in the smoking population to the evolution of attitudes toward smoking is exemplified by the shifts in smoking rates summarized in Table 3–4.[8] Per capita consumption of cigarettes plummeted by 25 percent in the 1980s. This was also the period of the greatest expansion in the public's willingness to take actions to restrict cigarette smoking.

Table 3–4 Principal economic aspects of smoking behavior

Year	Cigarettes per capita	Price per package ($avg.)	Taxes as a percent of retail price (median)	Cigarette smoker percentage	Former cigarette smoker percentage
1970	2,534	.39	46.8	36.7	17.9
1980	2,821	.63	33.1	32.6	20.6
1985	2,501	1.05	30.8	29.8	24.4
1989	2,156	1.44	26.4	NA	NA

Source: Tobacco Institute (1989), p. 6 (cigarettes per capita), and for price per package and tax percentage—p. 83 (1970), p. 93 (1980); and U.S. Department of Commerce (1989), p. 119 (smoking percentages).

A similar pattern is exhibited with respect to the smoking rates in the population. Whereas 37 percent of the population smoked in 1970, by 1985 this fraction had dropped to 30 percent. The fraction of former smokers in the population has also escalated, as 5 percent more of the population regarded themselves as being former smokers in 1985 than in 1970.

If one were considering these trends only in terms of the decrease in smoking that has taken place, they would be impressive. However, the extent of the shift in public attitudes toward smoking has been much greater than the statistics indicate. In particular, if there had not been such a reversal in public attitudes toward cigarettes, then the rates of smoking in the 1970s and 1980s would have continued to reflect an increase in smoking rates.

Figure 3–1 illustrates the long-run trends in per capita cigarette consumption throughout this century. The three cigarette warning eras are indicated as well. The patterns are not entirely smooth because a variety of economic and social factors are at work. The changing price of cigarettes, the shift in composition of the population, cyclical influences, and other cigarette risk-information events, and many other influences also will determine cigarette consumption, as they would for other commodities. Cigarette consumption, for example, declined in the early 1930s as a result of the Great Depression. Nevertheless, the long-run patterns of smoking are unmistakable.

The main test for the effect of antismoking policies is not their effect on the level of consumption, but whether they shift the consumption trend from the level that would otherwise have prevailed. In particular, what would smoking

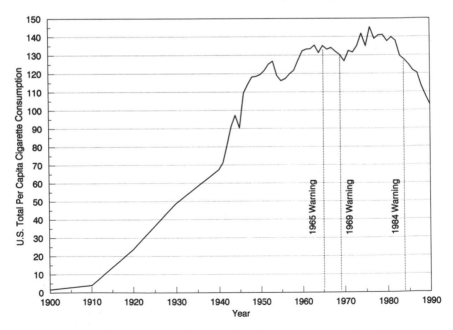

Figure 3–1 Trends in U.S. total per capita cigarette consumption, 1900–1989. *Source:* Tobacco Institute (1991), p. 6.

rates have been in the absence of the risk-information efforts? The patterns in Figure 3–1 illustrate how the rising per capita consumption of cigarettes in the first half of the century became halted, after which there was a relatively flat consumption period, followed by the current era of decline. The strong upward consumption trend had been reversed, reflecting a stark drop in the consumption patterns.

Until the early 1960s there was a fairly steady increase in per capita cigarette consumption. The temporary dip in the 1950s appears to be attributable to several factors. The postwar baby boom inflated the population base that is used to determine overall per capita cigarette consumption, although adult per capita consumption dropped as well. Smoking rates were also depressed by the publication of the 1953 Sloan-Kettering report linking smoking and lung cancer and by the widespread public discussion of the smoking-cancer risk at that time.[9] The 1960s and the 1970s marked a period of fairly stable smoking trends, which displayed a very slight increase from the level at the beginning of the 1960s. However, by the late 1970s and thereafter there was a steady decline in the rate of cigarette consumption.

The increasing price of cigarettes indicated in Table 3–4 no doubt contributed in part to this decline in smoking. However, the more important influence is clearly the shifting public attitudes toward the attractiveness of smoking as a consumption activity, which also includes the intensified public perception of the risk.

The different eras of hazard warnings also are related to the decline in smoking. The year 1965 marked the congressional passage of a bill requiring all cigarette packages to bear a warning by 1966. The influential government report on smoking issued in 1964 and the public discussion it generated also were important influences at that time. The second smoking warning was introduced in 1969, and the series of rotating warnings in 1984 is also indicated.

In every case the warnings were accompanied by a drop in smoking rates, although the extent of the decrease in the level of smoking in the mid-1960s does not appear to be particularly great. Moreover, there is no evidence of a discontinuous break in the smoking trend in 1984. The absence of identifiable drops in smoking rates is not a sign of a lack of impact since what matters is the observed decline in smoking rates from what they would have been in the absence of information. The main effect of the wave of information appears to have been that smoking rates became stabilized, whereas previously they had been following an upward trajectory. The net change in smoking rates from their expected level appears to have been substantial.

Major smoking events other than the advent of warnings also should be noted. In 1971 the ban on cigarette advertising on television and radio began, shortly after the new hazard-warning language (passed by Congress in 1969 and implemented in 1970) was required to be on cigarettes. The removal of smoking ads from television and radio was accompanied by the end of antismoking messages provided under the Fairness Doctrine. This compounding of simultaneous events makes it difficult to distinguish responsibility for the drop in cigarette consumption around 1970. This era was not exceptional in terms of the number of smoking-related events that might be influential.

None of these hazard warnings appears to have been a critical event that dramatically altered the trend in smoking rates. Nor was there a precipitous drop in smoking rates immediately after the landmark 1964 smoking report, although clearly this report had a substantial long-term influence. The impression conveyed by Figure 3–1 is quite consistent with econometric efforts to isolate the effect of hazard warnings. Smoking rates have shifted downward for a variety of reasons related to the social status of smoking and the intensified public perception of the risk. Even complex statistical studies directed at disentangling specific influences on smoking trends have not met with success.[10]

A variety of econometric studies have documented these shifts in smoking trends and their broad relationship to various information dissemination efforts. Hamilton (1972) found that the "health scare" with respect to cigarettes depressed cigarette consumption during the 1953–1970 period. The U.S. Federal Trade Commission report by Ippolito, Murphy, and Sant (1979) concluded that per capita consumption of cigarettes was depressed after the 1964 smoking report and after the 1953 tabulation of tar and nicotine levels in *Consumer Reports*. The FTC also concluded that there was a more gradual response to the 1964 cigarette warnings, as per capita consumption of cigarettes dropped by 3.5 percent from 1964 to 1975. However, there is no evidence that this decline intensified when the antismoking commercials were aired in 1968–1970. Warner (1989) concluded that in the absence of the antismoking campaign, including among other events the issuance of the Surgeon General's report, cigarette consumption in 1987 would have been 79 to 89 percent higher than the levels that occurred.[11] In the paper by Schneider, Klein, and Murphy (1981) that corrected many of the econometric problems in the earlier literature, the authors found there was a decline in cigarette consumption following both the 1953 report by the American Cancer Society and the British Medical Research Council's report on the higher death rates for smokers. There was also a decline in smoking rates following the 1964 smoking report. Finally, in their study of the Federal Communications Commission's Fairness Doctrine pertaining to the airing of antismoking messages from 1967 to 1971, Lewit, Coate, and Grossman (1981) found little or no impact on the total quantity of cigarette smokers, although there may have been a negative effect on the teenage smoking participation rate. McAuliffe (1988) found even weaker influences, as he could identify no significant effect of either the removal of the Fairness Doctrine or the cigarette advertising ban.

The central theme of these studies is that various government efforts to influence the amount of risk information that individuals have about cigarettes have lowered cigarette demand. However, it is not possible to disentangle the specific role that can be assigned to each particular form of policy intervention. In every case there were a number of contemporaneous events that complicate efforts to estimate the effects of specific policies; we can conclude, however, that the total dissemination of information in these time periods has resulted in a temporal shift in smoking trends.

One major contributor to the decreased level of smoking is not simply that fewer people start to smoke but also that many people who once smoked have quit smoking. Although 50 million Americans continue to smoke, half of all

American adults who once smoked have quit, and overall there are 38 million former smokers in the U.S. population.[12] Figure 3–2 indicates the trends in the quit ratio, which is the ratio of the percentage of individuals who are former cigarette smokers relative to the percentage of people who have ever smoked cigarettes. For the entire population, the quit ratio rose dramatically from 1965 to 1987, as it increased from just under 30 percent to almost 45 percent. Rates of smoking cessation are clearly at an all-time high.

Differences in the quit ratio reflect the changing educational composition of the smoking population. In 1966 the quit ratio for college graduates was 10 percent greater than for the entire population. By 1987 this difference had increased to over 14 percent. The quit ratio for all population groups has risen substantially over the past two decades, particularly for college graduates.

This is the type of response one would expect to observe. One possibility is that the college-educated may have obtained more information pertaining to the risk, leading to higher risk perceptions. However, this need not be the case for the observed results to hold true. Even if the effect on risk perceptions is the same for all age-groups, we would predict a stronger reaction on the part of the college-educated because the value that individuals attach to health hazards will be greater for this group. In particular, the valuation of risks to one's health status increases proportionally with one's income,[13] so that any given change in the

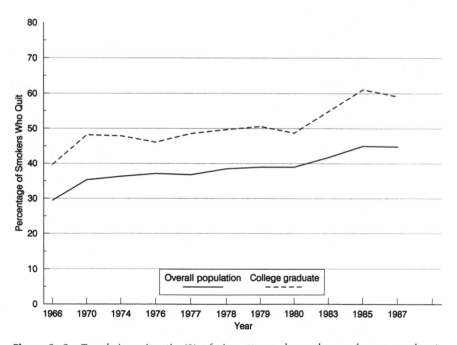

Figure 3–2 Trends in quit ratio (% of cigarette smokers who are former smokers), 1965–1987, age 20 and over. *Source:* U.S. Department of Health and Human Services (1990), p. 592.

perceived probability of an adverse health outcome will have a greater impact on the college-educated than on those whose lifetime earnings are less.

This phenomenon is not restricted to smoking. As we will document in Chapter 5, the same kinds of job risks that many white-collar workers would find unacceptable are in fact integral components of blue-collar occupations. A major reason for this difference stems from the role that individual wealth has in influencing one's attitudes toward risk. The evidence in Chapter 5 will indicate that the same kinds of individuals who choose not to wear seat belts and choose to smoke also are more willing to accept risky jobs. Thus, there are systematic differences in attitudes toward risk that stem from the valuations one attaches to health status, and these valuations are strongly correlated with income level.

In addition, the social controversy pertaining to smoking clearly affects its acceptability within one's sphere of activities. If one is college-educated, a greater preponderance of one's coworkers and friends will be nonsmokers than if one had only a high school education. Due to the increased societal concern about secondhand smoke and the social acceptability of smoking more generally, the pressures to quit smoking will clearly be greater for the college-educated than for those less educated. Irrespective of the underlying mechanism driving the increased quit ratio, it is clear that there has been a dramatic shift in the societal smoking rate.

There is little question that there has been a significant downward shift in smoking behavior over the past two decades and that this shift has been contemporaneous with the various informational events that have taken place. Unfortunately, it is difficult to isolate the causal factors involved because the introduction of hazard warnings has been accompanied by other events such as reports by the Surgeon General and widespread media publicity. In short, we do not have a pure experiment.

Because of the complications that have limited past investigations of time series analyses of smoking behavior, the focus of this volume will be on cross-sectional evidence. In particular, we will explore how various aspects of risk perceptions alter smoking behavior. What we will not be able to ascertain is which particular factors have influenced the development of these risk perceptions. As the review of the public opinion trends in the previous sections indicated, there was no single event to which these changing public perceptions can be traced. Instead, there has been a shift in public attitudes that has been uneven but nevertheless persistent for as long as data on public perceptions are available.

CONCLUSION

Trends in public opinion poll data suggest that there is increasing prevalence in the awareness of potential smoking risks. These findings, and particularly the pattern of substantial increases in risk perception over the past three decades, suggest that the various forms of cigarette risk information efforts that have been undertaken have succeeded in fostering greater awareness of these risks. Moreover, other aspects of smoking such as the risks posed by secondhand smoke have clearly become a prominent concern among the citizenry and policymakers.

The establishment of smoking risks in the public's view is not surprising. Smoking hazards have long received considerable media attention; smoking has been the subject of a substantial public debate and a diverse array of informational initiatives. Moreover, the risks implied by the early smoking warnings were of the same order of magnitude as the assessed risks posed by cigarettes. The presence of widespread risk perceptions is consistent with other evidence in psychology and economics on the character of risk perceptions and the nature of response to risk information.

Awareness of risks does not imply, however, that risk perceptions are accurate or that we should pronounce informational efforts a success. In subsequent chapters we will explore the character of risk perceptions and their impact on smoking behavior in greater detail.

NOTES

1. See Tate (1989), p. 108.

2. James B. Duke was the principal benefactor of Duke University. It is noteworthy that by 1991 Duke University had banned smoking in its medical center, in classrooms, at basketball games, and in many other campus buildings.

3. See Tate (1989), p. 110.

4. See Tate (1989), pp. 107–108.

5. U.S. Federal Trade Commission (1981), pp. 3–28.

6. This research was done jointly with Anil Gaba, professor at Institut Europeen D'Administration des Affaires (INSEAD), Fontainebleau, France.

7. U.S. Department of Health and Human Services (1989), p. 198.

8. For a further discussion of smoking trends, see Schelling (1986, 1988).

9. *Consumer Reports* and *Reader's Digest*, for example, published prominent articles on smoking hazards in these years; U.S. Department of Health and Human Services (1989), p. 658.

10. See, for example, Hamilton (1972) and Schneider, Klein, and Murphy (1981). For further review of this evidence, see U.S. Department of Health and Human Services (1989).

11. Earlier, Warner (1977) had estimated a 20 to 30 percent reduction in smoking in 1975 due to the antismoking campaign.

12. U.S. Department of Health and Human Services (1990), p. i.

13. See Viscusi and Evans (1990) for documentation.

4

Smoking Risk Perceptions

Individuals face a multitude of risks in their lives. For the most part, these risks arise because of particular actions individuals have taken and consumption decisions they have made. The hazards associated with transportation, work, and food consumption are among these risks, as few personal activities are risk-free. Some of these risks are known to those who bear them; others are not. For risks traded in a market context, the degree to which the risks are the result of a voluntary choice will hinge on individual knowledge of the risk.

The adequacy of smoking risk perceptions has long been a cornerstone of public policy with respect to smoking. The assumption of the American judicial system has been that smoking risks are not hidden. In its *Restatement of the Law of Torts* (Second), the American Law Institute observed:

> The articles sold must be dangerous to an extent beyond that which would be contemplated by the ordinary consumer who purchases it, with the ordinary knowledge common to the community as to its characteristics. Good whiskey is not unreasonably dangerous merely because it will make some people drunk, and is especially dangerous to alcoholics; but bad whiskey, containing a dangerous amount of fusel oil, is unreasonably dangerous. Good tobacco is not unreasonably dangerous merely because the effects of smoking may be harmful; but tobacco containing something like marijuana may be unreasonably dangerous.[1]

A number of unsuccessful court cases have recently challenged the adequacy of smokers' risk perceptions, and the extent to which individuals are aware of the risks posed by smoking is an obviously central concern in assessing the adequacy of market decisions.[2]

This chapter utilizes detailed data on individual risk perceptions and smoking behavior to investigate cigarette smoking as a potentially risky consumption activity.[3] In particular, to what extent do individuals have accurate perceptions of the risk? The literature reviewed in Chapter 2 indicates that important biases in risk perception are a frequent occurrence and that the direction of this bias may vary.[4] Do these errors in perception influence smoking behavior, or do smokers selectively ignore the bad information they have about smoking behavior? The character of this behavior is pertinent not only to the debate over smoking but also to the broader debate over the economics of cognitive dissonance.[5] In this chapter we will explore the pattern of smoking risk estimation using detailed data pertaining to lung cancer risk perceptions as well as data on mortality risks and life expectancy. Systematic biases in these risk perceptions are of policy interest as well, since ideally hazard warnings for cigarettes should foster more accurate risk perceptions.

The overall character of the results is that the level of lung cancer risk perceptions is very high. All segments of the population have substantial lung cancer risk assessments. The risk perceptions for the total mortality-risk and life-expectancy effects of smoking are also quite high. The most overestimated risk is lung cancer, which reflects the substantial publicity targeted at this class of hazards.

THE DATA BASE AND THE EMPIRICAL FRAMEWORK

Data Overview

Since the structure of the subsequent empirical analysis is dictated in large part by the nature of the data, let us consider the structure of the principal data base that will be used to explore smoking decisions in this and subsequent chapters. In September 1985 a New York survey research firm, Audits & Surveys, undertook a national telephone survey to ascertain the character of individual attitudes toward smoking and the nature of their risk perceptions.[6] The sampling procedure involved use of over 400 phone banks to call individuals nationwide, where the sampling was in proportion to the number of working residential phones in each stratum of the sample. To ensure a representative sample, the stratification was first performed by region (the four U.S. Census regions), which were then stratified into metropolitan and nonmetropolitan areas. The regional breakdown of the sample appears in Table 4–1.

Once making contact with a home, a random selection device was used to determine which household participant would be interviewed, where participation was restricted to persons age 16 or older. In particular, the interviewer asked the respondent a series of questions concerning the ages of the different family members, which established a comparable basis for ordering all households. Once this ordering was established, the preferred respondent was selected using a random selection procedure. This process continued until the interviewer had selected a respondent who was home.

The age distribution of the sample appears in Table 4–1. Just over half of the sample is in the large middle-aged cohort from age 22 to 45 (AGE22–45 dummy variable—d.v.), one-tenth are in the age 16–21 groups (AGE16–21 d.v.), and the remainder are over age 45 (AGE46+ d.v.) Under half of the sample consists of males (MALE d.v.), and the average household size is 2.2 (HOUSEHOLD SIZE).

The interview procedure was as follows. After informing the individual answering the phone that this survey was for "a study about cigarette smoking" and selecting the survey respondent from the household, the interviewer administered the questionnaire included in Appendix A. The interviewer first ascertained the respondent's overall reaction to cigarettes. This open-ended memory recall approach has proven to be an instructive technique for assessing the saliency of

Table 4–1 Sample characteristics

Variable	Mean (standard deviation)
AGE16–21 (Age 16–21 d.v.)	0.113
	(0.316)
AGE22–45 (Age 22–45 d.v.)	0.512
	(0.500)
AGE46+ (Age 46 or older d.v.)	0.368
	(0.482)
MALE	0.366
	(0.482)
HOUSEHOLD SIZE	2.193
	(0.983)
Regional dummy variables	
Northeast metro	0.170
	(0.376)
Northeast nonmetro	0.042
	(0.201)
North central metro	0.178
	(0.382)
North central nonmetro	0.086
	(0.280)
South metro	0.187
	(0.390)
South nonmetro	0.129
	(0.335)
West metro	0.169
	(0.374)
West nonmetro	0.039
	(0.195)
Variable	
RISK	0.426
	(0.269)
SMOKER	0.250
	(0.433)
FORMER SMOKER	0.248
	(0.432)
Sample size	3,119

taste-related factors and risk-related concerns in a manner that does not bias subsequent responses.[7] The question is asked before the lung cancer risk-perception question so that respondents are not alerted to the focus of the survey.[8] This approach elicits individual product attitudes without biasing responses by asking a series of questions highlighting the purpose of the survey (creating demand effects, i.e., the respondent giving the answer that he or she believes the interviewer wishes to hear) or increasing the salience of particular factors by mentioning these concerns in previous questions.

The survey then determined which of several statements the individual had heard about cigarettes (e.g., "cigarette smoking is bad for a person's health, but not dangerous") in an effort to ascertain the character of the respondent's prior information. The survey then ascertained the respondent's perception of lung cancer risks, which has long been viewed as a prominent and substantial potential hazard of cigarettes.

Obtaining meaningful survey responses regarding individuals' risk perceptions is not a straightforward task since one could ask for a probability, a number of deaths for a base population, or a rating on a risk scale shown to the respondents. For a phone interview, visual risk scales are infeasible. The approach used was to ascertain the lung cancer risk per 100 smokers: "Among 100 cigarette smokers, how many of them do you think will get lung cancer because they smoke?" As is discussed in Viscusi and Magat (1987), this approach of using a base population reference point is a more readily understood method for eliciting probabilistic information than dealing with probabilities or fractions explicitly. The sensitivity of the results to question formats will be explored later in the section on "Estimation of the Determinants of Risk Perceptions."

The wording of the question pertains to the risk to a group of smokers, not necessarily oneself. It may be that there is a discrepancy between the perceived risk to others and the perceived risk to oneself, should one choose to smoke.[9] Within the context of a telephone survey, it is unlikely that changes in question wording could reliably disentangle these influences. Asking smokers about a probability poses the question in probabilistic terms rather than the more readily understood form of a specific number out of 100 smokers. Such a question about personal risks would also not be pertinent to the nonsmoking population. Rather than explore such refinements in eliciting risk perceptions, the primary test for respondents' degree of belief in their stated risk perceptions will be whether these risk assessments influence smoking behavior.

After the individual's response to the lung cancer question is divided by 100, one obtains the lung cancer probability (RISK), which averaged .43 for the sample. Because of the central importance of the risk perception variable to the analysis, the empirical investigation is restricted to the 3,119 individuals for whom values of RISK were not missing. If the nonrespondents differ markedly from those who answer the risk-perception question, the result could be that the actual perceived risk in the population is distorted. This phenomenon, known as selection bias, is not always present in situations of incomplete responses. Moreover, we can do more than simply note the problem since econometricians have developed statistical methods to assess the importance of selection bias in a particular context. Chapter 6 explores the consequences of this selection problem in detail and presents results that take the influence of the possible selectivity bias into account. The principal implication of these findings is that there is no major effect of the sample selection on the results.

The survey addressed lung cancer risks but did not include information on all components of smoking risks. For example, one would have liked to have had information on the mortality assessments from lung cancer, not simply assessed lung cancer rates. My subsequent surveys, discussed later in this chapter, did address the cancer mortality risk component, yielding estimates similar to those for the overall lung cancer risk.

More importantly, there are other mortality and morbidity risks associated with smoking, including heart disease, strokes, and emphysema, and these are not included in the survey data. These risks also will be addressed using a more detailed data base. The perspective afforded by the Audits & Surveys data set will be limited to the link between lung cancer risk perceptions and smoking behavior. The manner in which this partial coverage affects the estimation procedure and the interpretation of the results will be indicated at appropriate junctures.

The other variables of interest are the individual's smoking status, in particular, whether the respondent is a current cigarette smoker (SMOKER d.v.), a former cigarette smoker (FORMER SMOKER d.v.), or has never smoked cigarettes. The smoking fraction is a bit below the national average of 32 percent,[10] which is not unexpected given the overrepresentation of women in a sample based on telephone interviews.

INDIVIDUAL PERCEPTIONS OF LUNG CANCER RISKS

The central focus of this book is on perceptions of smoking risks and the linkage of these perceptions to smoking behavior. The nature of these risk perceptions has long been a matter of policy controversy. The government has mandated a series of increasingly stringent on-product warnings so as to increase the perceived risk, and much of the impetus for societal concern with smoking stems from the possibility that smokers may be making uninformed choices.[11]

To the extent that there is evidence in the literature of inadequate smoking risk perceptions, it has been based on studies that did not utilize meaningful risk questions. For example, the Federal Trade Commission (1981, pp. 3–5) concluded that the stronger series of rotating warnings initiated in 1984 was needed since many smokers did not believe that smoking is "hazardous" or "causes cancer."

Past survey approaches that led to such conclusions are deficient in at least one of the following three ways. First, they often deal with statements for which the implied risk level is unclear. What level of risk is sufficient for an activity to be classified "hazardous"? Such risk thresholds are undefined and may vary greatly across respondents.[12] Second, the questions posed often treat risks that are probabilities as if they were nonstochastic. It is not correct to state that smoking "causes cancer" since this wording implies a certain link, when the true relationship is probabilistic. Third, individuals may not give correct responses to quiz questions on cigarette smoking trivia (e.g., what fraction of lung cancer is caused by cigarette smoking?), but this is not a fundamental concern.[13] Even if the respondent does not know the total role of lung cancer in society, he or she may know the incremental risks of smoking. What is at issue is not the correctness of the components of individual knowledge, but rather whether the overall risk judgments that result from this knowledge are accurate.

The RISK variable analyzed here consequently represents a considerable improvement over the smoking literature in terms of providing a meaningful risk measure. To assess the extent of bias in RISK perceptions, one must make some judgment regarding the "true" lung cancer risk level. Otherwise, we will have no reference point for assessing possible biases in risk perception. For concreteness, I will take the prevailing government views regarding the risks of smoking as the scientific standard. In particular, I will accept at face value the assessments of the risks of cigarette smoking that appear in the annual reports of the Surgeon General. The focus of the book consequently will be on how well individuals perceive and act upon the risks as they are characterized in these official government documents.

Use of this reference point does not necessarily imply acceptance of the estimates that have appeared in these reports. For example, there continues to be debate over whether some of the assessed differences in risk fully account for the multiple variables determining the risk. To what extent are cases of lung cancer caused by cigarette smoking as opposed to living in an urban area or working on a hazardous job?

The existing gaps in our knowledge may account for the fact that the annual reports exercise caution and do not state a specific risk level for cigarettes. There are voluminous tallies of illnesses and deaths from different populations, but readers will not find the Surgeon General or other leading government officials assigning specific probabilities to various outcomes of cigarette smoking, such as lung cancer and heart disease.

This reluctance to make specific probabilistic assessments is not because of a complete lack of information for doing so. Indeed, in this chapter I will construct such an assessment using information pertaining to the government's total of smoking-related diseases and the size of the smoking population. However, in all likelihood the underlying uncertainties in the scientific evidence have led policymakers to avoid assigning any specific risk level to cigarettes.[14]

These uncertainties do not imply that the research pertaining to smoking risks is particularly flawed. For almost any long-term risk there is a controversy regarding the extent of the causality and the nature of the dose-response relationship.[15] Problems in assigning causality are the norm in cases of toxic torts. Estimates of the number of job-related cases of cancer linked to asbestos vary by a factor of 10.[16] Similarly, there have been widely conflicting scientific judgments regarding the ailments of Vietnam veterans exposed to Agent Orange and the cancer cases of Woburn, Massachusetts, residents exposed to groundwater contamination from toxic pollutants.

Whenever we are dealing with a situation involving long-term health risks that are not signature diseases capable of being linked to particular actions or consumption decisions, risk assessments become imprecise. Long-term health hazards are particularly complex to assess because of the long gestation period before the effect of the risk exposure becomes apparent. Moreover, throughout the course of these decades there are thousands of individual decisions and exposures that also influence the ultimate health outcome. In many cases one cannot even generate reliable risk assessments so as to assign probabilistic causation. The best that can be done in the smoking context is to determine whether individual decisions under uncertainty are consistent with the best available scientific evidence at the time.

One might argue that because of the ambiguity we should err on the side of caution. In particular, we should forgo consumption activities that pose uncertain risks and avoid the unknown. Doing so is not typically a sensible strategy and will in fact lead to greater expected deaths and expected health losses than if we based our decisions on the level of the risk, not its precision. If we were to avoid an activity that posed a 1/1,000 risk of cancer that was uncertain and instead pursued an activity that posed a 2/1,000 risk of cancer that was known with precision because of our desire to avoid ambiguity, then we will in fact be putting ourselves at greater expected risk. We should always attempt to acquire information about the hazards in an effort to refine our risk assessments, and once we obtain this information we should maximize our expected welfare, treating "hard" and "soft" probabilities the same.[17] We should not in effect lie to ourselves about the expected consequences because of our aversion to the unknown.

Similarly, we should not make the opposite error of engaging in potentially risky consumption activities simply because the scientific evidence remains imprecise. We cannot dismiss hazards as being unimportant simply because conclusive scientific evidence has not been developed. The magnitude of some risks may never be resolved, but this does not imply that they are not of consequence. In the interim we must make decisions that will affect our lives in often consequential ways. In making these decisions we should utilize the best information available and act on these assessments.

Judgments of smoking risks are difficult to make since the scientific evidence is imprecise, and the scientific results are based largely on overall fatality risks of smokers as opposed to the specific contribution of cigarettes to lung cancer. Since cigarettes smoked in earlier decades had a much stronger tar and nicotine content than those smoked in the survey year 1985[18], and since smokers are more likely to engage in a variety of life-endangering pursuits, the evidence on estimated lung cancer risk levels may be biased upward.

Even after abstracting from this issue of the changing cigarette, there remains the issue of selecting a risk level for judging the accuracy of the lung cancer risks perceptions. There are two possible reference points. The first is the risk level believed to prevail at the time of the survey in 1985. Do the respondents have accurate beliefs that reflect the state of scientific knowledge at that time? An alternative approach is to ask whether these beliefs also reflect subsequent scientific knowledge and what is now believed to be the scientific truth. Imposing such a standard retroactively is an inappropriate standard for judging the soundness of earlier decisions. However, this more recent reference point is useful in determining whether the decisions based on previous knowledge continue to reflect the current estimate of the risks. The potential for a shift in societal risk perceptions accompanying the scientific knowledge should also be recognized.

The calculation of the risk probability associated with smoking is governed by both the number of adverse health outcomes and the size of the smoking population. Consider first the numerator of the risk calculation—the number of adverse health outcomes. Throughout the 1980s estimates of the total annual lung cancer mortality due to smoking were in the range of 93,000.[19] In 1991 some scientists increased this estimate to 117,000 annually.[20]

The other component of the risk probability is the denominator—the size of the population at risk. The number of smokers in 1985 was 52.9 million.[21] However, the risks of lung cancer and other smoking deaths occur with a lag. Recognition of this lag has little effect on the size of the smoking population, since the increase in the size of the total population is offset by the decline in the prevalence of smoking. In 1965, for example, there were 53.4 million smokers.[22] To make the total smoker number comparable with the health outcome measure, it must be in annual terms. This is done using a sensitivity analysis in which the lifetime smoking range is from thirty to sixty years. The upper end of this range is consequently excessively long, leading to a smaller annual smoking population and a higher estimate of the risk than is likely to be posed.

The result of these calculations is that the lung cancer death risk based on mid-1980s data is .05 to .10 per year. Using 1991 estimates and imposing this scientific knowledge retroactively leads to a lung cancer risk range of .06 to .125, which is not much greater. In the subsequent discussion, .05 to .10 will be the principal reference point used for assessing the accuracy of the survey responses.

In recognition of the uncertainty regarding the "true lung cancer risk" reference point, a sensitivity analysis will be performed using these two different reference points. These "true lung cancer risk" levels are primarily an expositional device for putting the empirical results in perspective. A change in the reference risk level to .20, for example, would alter the implications of the results very little. However, an increase in the risk level to a figure such as .60, which is well out of line with any risk estimates in the literature—even for all mortality risks from cigarettes—would necessitate a change in the nature of the discussion.

The distribution of lung cancer risk perceptions for the full sample and for smokers appears in Table 4–2. There is some clustering of responses around salient risk levels, such as .25 and .50, but the direction of bias imparted by such rounding is unclear. The population at large views the lung cancer risk from smoking as almost a 50–50 proposition, as the average value of RISK is .43. The levels differ by smoking status, with smokers having a lower risk assessment.

Not only is there no evidence of a downward bias in risk perceptions on average, but few people underestimate the lung cancer risk. For the "true lung cancer risk" level .05, 5.2 percent of the full sample and 9.2 percent of the smokers underestimate the risk, and for a "true risk" of .10 the percentage underestimating the risk rises to 9.7 for the full sample and 14.4 percent for smokers. In each case, many more individuals overestimate the risk than underestimate it.

Moreover, because the "true" lung cancer risk levels are closer to 0 than 1, the magnitude of the possible overestimation is greater as well. Consider the results for a true risk value of .05. For the full sample, individuals who underestimate

Table 4–2 Distribution of lung cancer risk perceptions for cigarette smoking

Distribution of lung cancer risk perceptions (RISK)	Fraction with risk perceptions in interval	
	Full sample	Current smokers
RISK < .05	.052	.092
.05 ≤ RISK < .10	.046	.051
.10 ≤ RISK < .20	.117	.130
.20 ≤ RISK < .30	.136	.146
.30 ≤ RISK < .40	.090	.114
.40 ≤ RISK < .50	.052	.050
.50 ≤ RISK < .60	.239	.228
.60 ≤ RISK < .70	.070	.056
.70 ≤ RISK < .80	.084	.050
.80 ≤ RISK < .90	.042	.027
.90 ≤ RISK < 1.0	.041	.028
RISK = 1.0	.030	.026
Mean RISK	.426	.368
(standard error of mean)	(.005)	(.009)
Sample size	3,119	779

the risk do so by an average amount of .02, whereas individuals who overestimate the risk do so by .47. For the full sample, the extent of overestimation is over twenty times as great as the amount of underestimation, and the frequency of overestimation is over nine times as great. Individuals consequently are more prone to overestimation of the risk and err in their overestimation by a substantial amount.

The survey's focus on lung cancer risks limits our ability to generalize about other smoking risk perceptions, such as for cardiovascular disease and morbidity effects. As a result, any conclusions in this section relating to biases in risk perceptions pertain to lung cancer risks, not all components of smoking hazards. Since mortality risk perceptions are bounded from above by 1.0, clearly individuals cannot overassess all components of the smoking risk by as much as they do for lung cancer. Results from local surveys reported later in this chapter suggest that overall, smoking risk perceptions are greater than the lung cancer perceptions but not by an amount that is proportional to the underlying difference in the true risks.

Even if all other risk perceptions were zero, which they are not, the overassessment of lung cancer risks will have important implications for any assessment of the likelihood of market failure. In particular, the substantial overestimation of lung cancer risks may more than compensate for any underestimation of other risk components.

Table 4–3 Actual smoking risk ranges in 1985 and 1991

Survey year	Lung cancer mortality risk to smoker	Total mortality risk to smoker	Total mortality risk to society
1985	.05–.10	.16–.32	.21–.42
1991	.06–.13	.18–.36	.23–.46

The scientific evidence on the total mortality risks of smoking has evolved over the past decade but has not undergone any abrupt shifts.[23] Table 4–3 summarizes the risk ranges for different time periods based on the available scientific evidence in those years. Consider first the risk to smokers. Recognition of the total mortality risk, not just that from lung cancer, would boost the lifetime risk range to .16 to .32 based on evidence through 1988, and to .18 to .36 based on 1989 evidence. The total smoking mortality risk is consequently roughly triple the lung cancer mortality risk. The total attributable mortality estimates linked to smoking behavior, including fetal risks and secondhand smoke, lead to an estimated risk range of .21 to .42 in 1985 and .23 to .46 in 1991.

Private decisions will be based primarily on the private risks to the smoker. Some social risks, such as fetal damage, will clearly be of greater concern to smokers than will social risks to remote parties, so that the risks pertinent to individual smoker decisions may lie between the private and social risk levels. The available scientific evidence at the time of the survey is the most pertinent reference point for judging the rationality of risk beliefs in a limited-information world. Nevertheless, comparison of risk perceptions with the 1991 scientific evidence is useful, just as economists often utilize a perfect-information reference point for assessing the soundness of economic decisions.

The perceived lung cancer risk estimates of the sample members are above the midpoints of all of these total mortality risk ranges. Even if individuals ignored all other smoking risks, the substantial lung cancer risk beliefs would create a major deterrent to smoking behavior.

The finding that individuals overestimate lung cancer risks of smoking is quite consistent with the literature on highly publicized events.[24] Cigarettes are a highly publicized risk, as the potential hazards of smoking have been the subject of media coverage and substantial social pressures. The overestimation of the lung cancer risks in the presence of such substantial information does not indicate a failure in individuals' ability to learn, but rather reflects the character of the information provided, as these informational efforts have attempted to raise risk perceptions.

Risk Information and Risk Perception

A salient policy concern is the extent to which various forms of information have influenced patterns of risk perception. The survey included a question asking whether the respondent had heard various notions about cigarettes, some of which should raise the risk perception and others which should lower the perceived risk. These ideas appear in the first column of Table 4–4. Thus, for example, the interviewer asked respondents whether they had heard that cigarette smoking will most likely shorten their life or whether they had heard that cigarette smoking is dangerous to a person's health. The first two sets of smoking ideas pertain to kinds of adverse information the individual may have received, and the next two ideas pertain to defenses of cigarette smoking that might undercut risk perceptions.

In each case and for each smoking status group, two kinds of information are presented. First, I indicate whether the individual has heard a particular type of information (HEARD). Then for the group that has heard this information, I indicate the value of their lung cancer risk perception (RISK). The risk perceptions are consequently conditional on the receipt of particular types of information.

One implication of this table is that most of the population has heard virtually all of the things listed. Approximately 70 percent of the population has heard that cigarette smoking is dangerous to your health. The least frequently heard statement is that cigarette smoking is not bad for a person's health. Clearly, the potential adverse consequences of cigarettes are not a closely guarded secret.

It is equally striking that no matter what you have heard, your risk assessment is not much affected. Consider, for example, the results for the full sample. The range in terms of the values of risk perceptions based on what people have heard is from .419 to .426—a difference of less than .01. The range in responses is not statistically significant for any of the columns of results. Given the precision of the estimates with the large sample size, this invariance represents a very strong test, indicating that the kinds of information listed in this table have no significant effect on risk perceptions. There appears to be no new informational content in any of the four ideas expressed in the table, so that the determinants of risk

Table 4–4 Profile of groups who have heard ideas about cigarette smoking

	Fractions who have heard idea (HEARD), their risk perception (RISK), and standard error of mean risk							
	Full sample		Current smoker		Former smoker		Nonsmoker	
	HEARD	RISK	HEARD	RISK	HEARD	RISK	HEARD	RISK
Cigarette smoking will most likely shorten life	.634	.423 (.006)	.602	.365 (.012)	.656	.395 (.012)	.639	.465 (.008)
Cigarette smoking is dangerous to a person's health	.703	.422 (.006)	.680	.363 (.011)	.705	.399 (.012)	.713	.460 (.008)
Cigarette smoking is bad for a person's health but not dangerous	.627	.419 (.006)	.630	.356 (.012)	.642	.408 (.012)	.619	.458 (.008)
Cigarette smoking is not bad for a person's health	.567	.426 (.006)	.555	.362 (.013)	.571	.407 (.013)	.573	.466 (.009)

perceptions and variations in risk perceptions seem to be much more sophisticated than is captured by these simple statements. This is a pattern one would
expect in a situation in which individuals have already acquired substantial
information about a product.

ESTIMATION OF THE DETERMINANTS OF RISK PERCEPTIONS

The sources of smoking information affecting risk perceptions are quite diverse.
An individual utilizes his or her prior beliefs about smoking risks, information on
the smoking experiences of oneself or others, and information provided by the
media (including cigarette advertising) or through various government policies.
These are the factors that I include in a statistical model in which risk perceptions
are treated as a linear function of a variety of variables, such as respondent age.[25]
Other specifications of the risk-perception equation led to very similar results, so
the analysis will focus on the simple linear model.[26] This approach has the
advantage that it is based on a formal theory of rational (i.e., Bayesian) learning,
the details of which will be explored in Chapter 6. Since the RISK variable
pertains to lung cancer risks and not all risks of smoking, this equation provides
only a partial assessment of the determinants of all smoking risk perceptions.
Omission of these other risks does not bias the estimated influence of the determinants of lung cancer risk perceptions since this variable is the dependent
variable in the analysis.

Table 4–5 reports several specifications of the lung cancer risk-perception
equation in which different sets of variables are included so as to distinguish the
different influences at work. The estimated coefficients in Table 4–5 indicate
how much a unit charge in each variable would affect the assessed value of
RISK. For example, controlling for other influences, males assess RISK as being
.05 to .06 lower than do females.

Equation 1 in Table 4–5 includes only the background variables and regional
dummy variables, which reflect differences in experience and the character of
information that has been acquired. The youngest age-group (AGE16–21) has
higher risk perceptions, which is consistent with the smoking information the
youngest cohort has received, including a much higher fraction of high-risk
messages. The Surgeon General's efforts and the character of cigarette warnings
have become more stringent in recent years, and there has been a dramatic
increase in social pressure against smoking. One would have expected the younger respondents to be more heavily affected by the recent antismoking campaigns. Males have a significantly lower risk perception on average. This pattern
may reflect sex differences in attitudes toward risk or a difference in exposure to
smoking. Both the AGE16–21 and MALE coefficients remain strongly significant in all five specifications, so that these effects are not attributable to the
omission of other substantive variables.

Equation 2 of Table 4–5 adds a series of four variables that pertain to whether
the individual has heard different statements about cigarette smoking, thus capturing the role of various forms of information that has been received. In particu-

Table 4–5 Lung cancer risk assessment equations[a]

Independent variables	Coefficients (standard errors)		
	1	2	3
Intercept	0.4362[b]	0.4790[b]	0.5175[b]
	(0.0172)	(0.0242)	(0.0246)
AGE 16–21	0.0736[b]	0.0711[b]	0.0546[b]
	(0.0170)	(0.0170)	(0.0170)
AGE 22–45	0.0028	−0.0004	−0.0004
	(0.0104)	(0.0105)	(0.0104)
MALE	−0.0564[b]	−0.0556[b]	−0.0489[b]
	(0.0100)	(0.0100)	(0.0099)
HOUSEHOLD SIZE	0.0041	0.0039	0.0032
	(0.0050)	(0.0051)	(0.0050)
Ideas heard			
SHORTENS LIFE	—	−0.0079	−0.0084
		(0.0135)	(0.0134)
DANGEROUS TO HEALTH	—	−0.0237[b]	−0.0262
		(0.0140)	(0.0138)
BAD, NOT DANGEROUS	—	−0.0382[b]	−0.0360[b]
		(0.0135)	(0.0134)
NOT BAD FOR HEALTH	—	0.0089	0.0051
		(0.0133)	(0.0132)
PAST OR CURRENT SMOKER	—	—	−0.0681[b]
			(0.0097)
$\bar{R}^2$	.02	.02	.03

[a] Each equation also includes a series of seven regional dummy variables.
[b] Denotes coefficients that are statistically significant at the 5 percent level, one-tailed test.

lar, respondents were asked whether they had heard that "cigarette smoking will most likely shorten a person's life" (SHORTENS LIFE), "cigarette smoking is dangerous to a person's health" (DANGEROUS TO HEALTH), "cigarette smoking is bad for a person's health but not dangerous" (BAD, NOT DANGEROUS), and "cigarette smoking is not bad for a person's health" (NOT BAD FOR HEALTH).[27]

The four informational variables included in equation 2 of Table 4–5 have little effect on risk perceptions, which suggests that these statements have little informational content beyond what people already know. Two of the variables have coefficients that are not statistically significant, and the other two are of small magnitude. Somewhat surprisingly, the statement that is closest to the 1965 Surgeon General's warning (DANGEROUS TO HEALTH) is associated with a risk perception .02 lower than average. A somewhat greater negative discrepancy of −.04 is observed for BAD, NOT DANGEROUS. In each case the effect on risk perceptions is relatively small compared with the overall risk perception of .43.

The final equation 3 in Table 4–5 includes whether the respondent has ever smoked either in the past or at present.[28] Since this variable could potentially be endogenous with risk perceptions affecting the smoking experience variable, this possibility was tested formally and rejected.[29] Statistical tests indicate that one cannot reject the hypothesis that PAST OR CURRENT SMOKER is not endogenous. Moreover, the results in Chapter 6 indicate the overall performance of the risk perception equation estimated within the context of a simultaneous model of smoking decisions and risk perceptions yields similar results. Past smoking has the expected negative effect on risk perceptions, as a smoking history reduces the perceived RISK probability by .07.

It should be noted that the equations estimated have low explanatory power overall. If our concern were with predicting the risk perceptions of a particular person, these results would suggest that the equations provided an imprecise basis for doing so. What these results do suggest is that the individual differences in smoking risk perception cannot be readily accounted for by the four Ideas Heard variables or broad measures of demographic background.

Probability of Risk Underestimation

From a market failure standpoint, one's main concern is not with the overall level of risk perception but with the probability that these perceptions are below the "true risk." Thus, one could replace the dependent variable in Table 4–5 by the probability that the risk is underestimated. Such an assessment provides an insight into the character of an important cigarette risk component but of course will not address all other smoking-related risks.

Table 4–6 presents logit estimates of the risk underestimation equation using two different "true lung cancer risk" reference points—.05 and .10. The results are quite similar to the RISK perception equation. The YOUNG sample members are less likely to underestimate the risk, and MALE sample members are more likely to underestimate the risk. Individuals with a smoking history are more likely to underestimate the risk, but the effect is fairly small.

It is particularly striking that none of the four informational variables has a statistically significant effect on risk underestimation. These results do not imply that knowledge is unimportant. Rather, they suggest that there is sufficiently widespread familiarity with the knowledge tested that this knowledge is uncorrelated with smoking risk perceptions.

ALTERNATIVE RISK QUESTION FORMATS: ARE THE FINDINGS ROBUST?

How one asks the risk-perception question can be of substantial consequence. Fischhoff and MacGregor (1983), for example, found that the fatality risk levels associated with various diseases varied substantially depending on how the question was posed. This sensitivity suggests that whatever risk perception question wording is chosen should be well understood by respondents. The death rate per

Table 4–6 Probability that individual underestimates the risk, logit model

	Coefficients (standard errors)			
	True risk = 0.05		True risk = 0.10	
Independent variables	1	2	3	4
Intercept	−2.9914^a	−4.0834^a	−2.3041^a	−3.0131^a
	(0.3121)	(0.4548)	(0.2286)	(0.3332)
YOUNG	−0.7860^a	−0.5142	−0.7429^a	−0.5468^a
	(0.3398)	(0.3462)	(0.2427)	(0.2470)
ADULT	−0.3560^a	−0.3083^a	−0.4290^a	−0.4003^a
	(0.1720)	(0.1737)	(0.1294)	(0.1308)
MALE	0.5794^a	0.4775^a	0.5622^d	0.4870^a
	(0.1647)	(0.1660)	(0.1236)	(0.1246)
HOUSEHOLD SIZE	−0.0840	−0.0739	−0.0395	−0.0300
	(0.0937)	(0.0911)	(0.0669)	(0.0678)
Ideas heard				
SHORTENS LIFE	—	−0.0671	—	0.0101
		(0.2214)		(0.1720)
DANGEROUS TO HEALTH	—	0.3614	—	0.2473
		(0.2290)		(0.1793)
BAD, NOT DANGEROUS	—	0.3667	—	0.2668
		(0.2306)		(0.1677)
NOT BAD FOR HEALTH	—	0.1263	—	−0.1208
		(0.2246)		(0.1670)
PAST OR CURRENT SMOKER	—	0.8601^a	—	0.6766^a
		(0.1807)		(0.1302)
Log likelihood	−615.16	−599.88	−968.83	−952.53

^{a}Denotes coefficients that are statistically significant at the 5 percent level, one-tailed test.

100 smokers is a natural question format, but one should ascertain that the reported risk beliefs do not change markedly with reasonable changes in question formulation.

Lung Cancer Perception Sensitivity Tests

Consider the average respondent who indicated that the lung cancer risk level was .43 when the risk question was expressed in terms of the risk per 100 smokers. Would these same respondents indicate a risk of 430 per 1,000 smokers? Similarly, if a telephone survey were replaced by a written questionnaire using a different kind of risk scale, would we elicit the same risk-perception results?

The procedure utilized in the Audits & Surveys data has much to recommend it. People can conceptualize the risk per 100 smokers easily, as it provides a natural way to think about probabilities. Moreover, it is easy to comprehend within the context of a telephone interview. All question formats are not of interest since clearly the results derived from a misleading or confusing question format may be different. However, legitimate variations of question structure should not be of major consequence if the original survey estimates are a reliable index of smoking risk beliefs.

Using a series of telephone surveys undertaken in 1990 and 1991 in the Durham, North Carolina, area, I explored the sensitivity of the risk responses to variations in the question formulation. First, to establish a baseline in terms of the representativeness of the 1990–1991 Durham sample as compared with the 1985 national sample, I first undertook a survey that repeated the original wording of the Audits & Surveys question. Fifty-three respondents who answered the question pertaining to the number among 100 smokers who would get lung cancer indicated an average risk of .41, which was not significantly different from the risk of .43 in the Audits & Surveys data.

For a different sample, I then altered the denominator in the question to ascertain how many among the 2 million cigarette smokers in North Carolina would get lung cancer because they smoke. Virtually no respondents processed this information and incorporated it in their response. Instead, most simply gave a response in percentage terms. An additional variation along the same lines is that I utilized a question that asked respondents how many among 1,000 cigarette smokers would get lung cancer because they smoke. Once again, the overwhelming majority of the respondents ignored this specific numerical information for the denominator of the risk assessment, and they simply responded in percentage terms. Within the context of a telephone survey, these results suggest that the approach of posing the risk in terms of the number of adverse outcomes to a group of 100 smokers is an easy way for respondents to conceptualize the probabilities involved. In the discussion below, I will also review sensitivity tests using a written survey in which we can place greater demands on the respondents in terms of the structure of the risk question.

The respondents to the Audits & Surveys questions indicated belief in a substantial risk to smokers of contracting lung cancer. However, these respondents may not necessarily have believed that all those adversely affected will die of lung cancer. An American Cancer Society survey that asked respondents about the probability of surviving lung cancer if it is "detected early" indicated that respondents had an overoptimistic belief regarding the survivability of lung cancer.[30] This survey was flawed because the wording of the question implied that there was the potential for constructive action. Moreover, even if respondents believed the health outcome to be nonfatal, from the standpoint of individual choice, risk perceptions will still play a substantial role if the perceived outcome is very undesirable.[31]

To examine the mortality issue more appropriately, I utilized the following risk question with a different sample of 206 respondents contacted from fall 1990 through spring 1991: "Among 100 cigarette smokers, how many of them do you think will die from lung cancer because they smoke?" Table 4–7 summarizes the responses by smoking status. The average risk assessment was .38, which was a bit lower than the overall lung cancer risk assessment of .41 yielded in the Durham, North Carolina, telephone survey. These differences were not statistically significant. The principal ramification of this result is that the assessed lung cancer fatality rate from smoking is very similar to the assessed lung cancer incidence rate.

Total Mortality Effects

All individuals who participated in the survey with the fatal lung cancer risk question were also given the following question to ascertain the overall smoking mortality rate: "Among 100 cigarette smokers, how many of them do you think will die from lung cancer, heart disease, throat cancer, and all other illnesses because they smoke?" The final column of Table 4–7 summarizes the responses to this question conditional on various smoking status variables. The average risk assessment of the total incremental smoking mortality rate is .54, which is 1.42 times as large as the assessed lung cancer mortality rate for the same sample. Respondents' assessed smoking mortality rate is two to three times as great as the actual total mortality risk from smoking.[32] Individuals consequently overassess the total mortality risks from cigarettes, but the extent of overestimation is less than that for lung cancer risk.

Such a decrease in the overestimation of risk is expected for two reasons. First, lung cancer risks have received the greatest attention for the longest period of time. The early antismoking efforts and the initial reports by the Surgeon General focused on lung cancer, and the risk continued to be the most prominent smoking hazard. A second influence that will tend to reduce the extent of overestimation of all smoking risks is that risk assessments must necessarily be bounded from above by 1.0. This constraint will tend to compress the overestimation of probabilities larger than the lung cancer risk level. The general spirit of the results is consistent with the lung cancer risk findings in that they

Table 4–7 Smoking fatility risk perceptions[a]

Sample	Mean (standard error of the mean)	
	Lung cancer fatality risk	Total smoking mortality risk
Full sample	.38 (.02)	.54 (.07)
Current smokers	.31 (.04)	.47 (.05)
Current nonsmokers	.40 (.02)	.56 (.03)
Former	.36 (.03)	.50 (.04)
Never	.42 (.03)	.59 (.03)

[a] Sample size = 206.

indicate substantial awareness of the risks of smoking that are not sensitive to the wording of the telephone survey.

The smoking mortality risk perceptions in Table 4–7 are conditional on smoking status and follow patterns similar to those in the national survey reported in Table 4–2. Current smokers assess the lung cancer fatality risk as being .31, which is .11 below the assessed risk by individuals who have never smoked. The overall smoking mortality risk perceptions vary similarly. Current smokers assess the total smoking mortality risk as being .47, whereas individuals who have never smoked assess it as being .59. Individuals with lower smoking risk perceptions are more likely to smoke.

These results also are not particularly sensitive to the information that individuals may have heard about smoking. Table 4–8 indicates the ideas that individuals may have heard about cigarettes for the sample of individuals who responded to the smoking mortality questions. The wording of these questions was identical to those questions reported in Table 4–4 for the Audits & Surveys data set. The five-year difference in the timing of the surveys and the utilization of a city such as Durham, North Carolina, which is located in a tobacco-producing region, may account for the striking difference in the information that people have heard about cigarettes. Ninety-nine percent of the respondents in the survey results in Table 4–8 had heard that cigarettes shorten life, and all of the respondents had heard that cigarettes are dangerous to one's health, whereas only two-thirds of the respondents to the 1985 survey had heard these statements. Similarly, a small minority of respondents had heard that cigarettes are not bad for a person's

Table 4–8 Risk information and smoking fatality risk perceptions[a]

Information heard	Overall frequency	Cancer fatality risk	Total smoking mortality risk
Cigarette smoking will most likely shorten life			
Have heard	.99	.48	.59
Have not heard	.01	.45	.50
Cigarette smoking is dangerous to a person's health			
Have heard	1.00	.48	.59
Have not heard	0.00	—	—
Cigarette smoking is bad for a person's health but not dangerous			
Have heard	.31	.43	.57
Have not heard	.69	.44	.60
Cigarette smoking is not bad for a person's health			
Have heard	.16	.33	.55
Have not heard	.84	.50	.601

[a]Sample size = 206.

health, and almost one-third had heard that cigarettes are bad but not dangerous, whereas a majority of the respondents in Table 4–4 had heard these statements. The information that individuals have heard about smoking does not appear to have great factual content, as the cancer fatality risk assessments and the overall smoking mortality risk assessments are not significantly different, irrespective of what the individual may have heard. The main exception is the final informational entry—cigarette smoking is not bad for a person's health—which may be a generally proxy for risk perceptions.

Duration of Life Lost

Even though individuals believe that the probability of death from smoking is high, they may err in their judgment regarding the timing of these deaths and the amount of life that will be lost. To address this issue, I developed a telephone survey question pertaining to the life-expectancy effects. For the responses to the question to be meaningful, respondents must have a good notion of what the magnitude of life expectancy at risk is for the reference-point demographic group. Without such information, the survey task becomes much more difficult, possibly tainting the validity of the responses. The wording of the question, which varied with the sex of the respondent, was as follows: "The average life expectancy for a 21-year-old male(female) is that he(she) would live for another 53(59) years. What do you believe the life expectancy is for the average male (female) smoker?" The question does not ask respondents to assess the life-expectancy loss to avoid biasing the results by mentioning the prospect of a "loss." One can compute the loss in life expectancy using the response to the question in conjunction with the sex-specific life-expectancy value.

Table 4–9 summarizes the assessed loss in life expectancy for different groups in a sample of 120 telephone respondents in Durham, North Carolina, who were

Table 4–9 Respondents' assessed life-expectancy loss due to smoking[a]

| | Mean (standard error of the mean) | | |
Sample	Males	Females	Total
Full sample	8.5	13.2	11.5
	(0.9)	(0.9)	(0.7)
Current smokers	6.9	10.9	9.0
	(1.2)	(3.0)	(1.7)
Current nonsmokers	9.1	13.7	12.3
	(1.2)	(0.9)	(0.7)
Former	6.5	13.2	10.8
	(2.4)	(1.6)	(1.1)
Never	10.8	13.9	13.0
	(1.1)	(1.1)	(0.8)

[a]Sample size = 120.

polled in 1991. Overall, the assessed life-expectancy loss from smoking is 11.5 years. The assessed loss in life expectancy ranges from 9.0 for current smokers to 13.0 for those who have never smoked. Females assess a greater life-expectancy loss than do males. This difference may largely reflect the fact that women have six more years of life expectancy that is at risk.

The life-expectancy loss estimates reflect the combined influence of the respondent's assessment of shift in the mortality distribution from smoking and the years of life lost at that age. Table 4–10 presents the life-expectancy loss value conditional on the respondent's assessed mortality risk level. As we move from the lowest mortality risk group (0–.20) to the highest group (.81–1.00), the assessed loss in life expectancy rises from 7.0 to 18.8 years. There is clearly a strong correlation between the life-expectancy loss responses and the assessed mortality risk levels, which provides a consistency test of the responses.

The degree of accuracy of the life-expectancy loss assessments is also a matter of concern. Is the assessed expected loss of life above or below the scientific estimates of the effect of smoking on the duration of life? The 1968 Report of the Surgeon General estimated the smoking-related loss in life expectancy among young men as being eight years for heavy smokers (over two packs a day) and four years for light smokers (less than half a pack per day).[33] More recent studies that have increased smoking mortality estimates also imply that the estimated loss in life expectancy is greater, but no comparable official figures for life-expectancy loss are available for the more recent period. The 1989 Report of the Surgeon General did, however, indicate that each person who dies of a smoking-related fatality loses approximately 20 years of life.[34] For smoking mortality rates in the range of .18 to .36 based on 1991 data, the estimated life-expectancy loss is 3.6 to 7.2 years, which is well below the survey estimates. Individuals' assessed life-expectancy loss is greater than the scientists' estimates of the

Table 4–10 Comparison of assessed life-expectancy loss and fatality risk of smoking[a]

Assessed mortality risk level (deaths/100 smokers)	Number in cell	Mean (standard error) assessed life-expectancy loss
0–20	25	7.0 (1.3)
21–40	18	8.3 (1.4)
41–60	35	12.3 (1.2)
61–80	32	13.8 (1.0)
81–100	10	18.8 (3.7)

[a]Sample size = 120.

loss attributable to smoking, so that this evidence is consistent with the risk-perception findings.

The estimated loss in life expectancy found in my 1991 survey is greater than that found in two studies using 1980 data. Hamermesh and Hamermesh (1983) estimated that white male smokers assessed their life-expectancy loss as four years, a result that they concluded was consistent with available scientific evidence at the time of their study. A 1980 Roper survey used by Ippolito (1987) and by Ippolito and Ippolito (1984) indicated that respondents assessed a life-expectancy loss of approximately 3.5 years.[35] These estimates are below those found in my sample for several reasons. These other surveys pertained to life-expectancy loss from a different base age level—30 years old (Roper survey) and respondent's own age (Hamermesh and Hamermesh—mean age of 43 for their sample), whereas my study used a common base of age 21 to assess the loss of life expectancy at the onset of smoking. It is this loss that is the counterpart to the scientists' assessments of the life-expectancy effects, not the loss at some later age. The risk-perception era in other studies was also a decade earlier, and these surveys provided no information to respondents concerning the amount of life expectancy at risk.

Risk Assessments with a Written Survey

The final variation of the results alters the risk question in several ways.[36] First, the context of the survey is not cigarette risks but food cancer risks more generally. Second, rather than utilizing a telephone survey, the results are based on a written questionnaire, making it possible to utilize more complex risk questions. Third, instead of using a base population of 100 smokers, the study uses both the population in the entire state as the reference point and a linear risk scale. Finally, the focus is on total smoking cancer deaths rather than the incidence of lung cancer cases.

The smoking risk perception scale was elicited through the chaining of two different risk questions. In particular, consumers were asked to rate the severity of the hazard warning indicating that the product contained a chemical known to cause cancer on a risk scale in which risks posed by cigarettes and saccharin products were the principal reference points. An alternative question established the risk in terms of the state's total population, and linking the two questions establishes a metric for the smoking risk. Because the respondents were a group of ninety-nine adults from the Chicago area, the reference state population was that of Illinois.

More specifically, the various risk ranges that the individual could select appear in Table 4–11. The respondents had to pick one of three risk ranges into which a product bearing the cancer warning discussed in Chapter 3 would fall. The first risk range was from a zero level of risk to that posed by one 12-ounce cola that contained saccharin. The second risk range was a risk from that posed by one cola drink containing saccharin to one pack of cigarettes, and the final risk range was from one to five packs of cigarettes. The fraction of respondents who put the cancer-causing chemical in the different risk ranges is given in the

Table 4–11   Risk assessment for the reference warning indicating that the product contains a chemical that causes cancer

Risk range	Fraction who put product in range	Score within range on a 10-point scale
1. Zero risk–one 12-oz. saccharin cola	.21	4.86
2. One saccharin cola–one pack of cigarettes	.44	4.27
3. One pack of cigarettes–five packs of cigarettes	.35	2.25

Source: Viscusi (1988), p. 307.

first column of results in Table 4–11. Overall, 44 percent of all the survey participants believed that a cancer-causing chemical posed a risk between that posed by a cola drink containing saccharin and one pack of cigarettes.

Respondents were then asked to rate the risk of the product within the range they had selected on a scale of one to ten, 10 being the highest risk rating. The average rating was 5 for respondents who picked the lowest risk range. Respondents who selected the "one saccharin cola to one pack of cigarettes" range had an average score of 4. For respondents selecting the high risk range of "1 to 5 packs of cigarettes," the average risk rating was 2.

We can infer the implied risk levels using the risk-range responses and the information regarding the risk equivalent of the reference chemical cancer warning. Overall, respondents indicated that the product with the reference cancer risk warning posed a risk equivalent to smoking .58 packs of cigarettes daily.[37]

The survey then ascertained how many of the 11 million Illinois residents using the reference product would be killed by consumption of the product. Their average response of 1,316,729 deaths per 11 million people indicated a death risk of .12. Thus, respondents viewed a fatality risk of .12 as equivalent to the risk posed by .58 packs of cigarettes. The implied death risk per pack is .21. Based on current population smoking rates, respondents' overall assessed average cancer death risk to a cigarette smoker with the average rate of cigarette consumption is consequently .33.[38] This estimate is of the same general magnitude as some of the highest estimates of the overall smoking mortality rate that have appeared in the literature. Given the less representative character of the food cancer warning study and the quite different survey approaches, these findings are quite similar to the results above. Establishing this linkage also suggests that the results in this chapter are likely to be reasonably robust with respect to variations in survey methodology that enable respondents to address probabilities in a meaningful manner.

CONCLUSION

To explore perceptions of smoking risks, I have used data based on six different survey approaches:

1. Lung cancer cases per 100 smokers (telephone),
2. Lung cancer cases per 1000 and per 2 million smokers (telephone sensitivity test),
3. Lung cancer deaths per 100 smokers (telephone),
4. Total deaths per 100 smokers (telephone),
5. Life expectancy loss (telephone), and
6. Linear risk scale and cancer death risk per 11 million state residents (written survey).

The similarity of the responses for different question formulations suggests that the empirical findings are not an artifact tied to some specific question phrasing.

The assessment of the role of lung cancer risks indicated that these risk perceptions were quite substantial and appear to be biased upward, which is consistent with psychological evidence on highly publicized risks. The lung cancer component of smoking risks has received the greatest attention, and not surprisingly the associated risk perceptions are relatively high. Evidence for lung cancer fatalities, overall smoking fatalities, and life-expectancy loss from smoking suggests that the risks of smoking are not underassessed. However, the extent of overestimation of the risk is much greater for lung cancer risks than for overall smoking mortality, as one would expect given the greater publicity this component of smoking hazards has received.

Despite the provision of extensive smoking information, individuals have biased perceptions, not accurate risk beliefs. These biases may reflect the character of societal information transfer and the social pressure against smoking. Recent antismoking efforts have included stronger on-product warnings. The warnings that were in place at the time of the national survey declared that "smoking causes lung cancer." Even the 1969–1983 warning that "cigarette smoking is dangerous to your health" conveys a very high risk. These warnings requirements have been coupled with an increasingly vigorous antismoking effort, including a campaign by the former Surgeon General for a "smoke-free society." The result has been high risk perceptions that reflect the character of the information provided and the manner in which individuals with limited cognitive abilities process the risk information they receive.

Perhaps the most important general lesson for risk communication is that risk information and media coverage serve primarily to raise risk perceptions. This role contrasts with the usual economic assumption that greater information necessarily fosters more accurate beliefs. In the next chapter we will explore how these perceptions affect the decision to smoke.

NOTES

1. Section 402A, comment i, American Law Institute (1965), pamphlet 2, p. 352.
2. See Crist and Majoris (1987).
3. Thus, this chapter is related more generally to the literature on the economics of the rationality of individual choice under uncertainty. Particularly pertinent contributions include Arrow (1982), Blomquist (1979), Camerer and Kunreuther (1989), Lucas (1986),

Peltzman (1973, 1975, 1987), Viscusi (1984, 1985a,b), Viscusi and Magat (1987), and Viscusi, Magat, and Huber (1987).

4. See, for example, Arrow (1982), Camerer and Kunreuther (1989), Combs and Slovic (1979), Fischhoff et al. (1981), Kahneman and Tversky (1979), Lichtenstein et al. (1978), Viscusi (1985a,b), and Viscusi and Magat (1987).

5. See Akerlof and Dickens (1982).

6. This survey was commissioned by the defense law firms in support of tobacco litigation efforts.

7. See Magat, Viscusi, and Huber (1988) for a detailed discussion of the memory recall technique.

8. Test surveys that omitted the smoking attitude and information heard questions yielded lung cancer risk responses that were not statistically different from those that included these questions. This robustness test was undertaken by the author using a Durham, North Carolina, telephone survey.

9. See Marsh (1985) and Chapter 4 of the U.S. Department of Health and Human Services (1989).

10. The U.S. average smoking percentage was 32.1 in 1983. See the U.S. Department of Commerce (1985), p. 119.

11. A review of these warnings and consumers' differing assessments of the relative risks implied by the warnings appears in Viscusi (1988).

12. As noted in Chapter 3, recent work by Anil Gaba and myself on workers' perceptions of whether jobs are "dangerous" indicates that the objective risk threshold for labeling a job "dangerous" declines with the level of education.

13. The U.S. Federal Trade Commission (1981), pp. 3–21, for example, notes that 60 percent of all smokers do not believe that cigarettes are the major cause of lung cancer. These questions address broad knowledge of risks in general, not the incremental risk attributable to smoking, which is the main matter of concern.

14. The scientific evidence for the risks posed by secondhand smoke is even more muddled. Some scientists claim that these risks are negligible, whereas others project substantial societal death risks arising from secondhand smoke.

15. See Viscusi (1991b), Brennan (1989), and Schuck (1986).

16. See Viscusi (1991b).

17. Indeed, if we have a sequence of trials, experimentation with the uncertain risk is desirable for any given mean risk level. This is the classic two-armed bandit problem.

18. U.S. Department of Health and Human Services (1983), p. 372.

19. In particular, risk estimates prevailing at the time of the survey indicated that there are 110,000 lung cancer deaths per year, 85 percent (or 93,500) of which are believed to be due to smoking (U.S. Department of Health and Human Services [1982], p. vi). This death rate represents a lung cancer risk of .0017 per year of smoking, that is, the number of lung cancer deaths divided by the number of smokers (U.S. Department of Commerce [1985], p. 19). More recent estimates of the lung cancer death risks from smoking are of a similar magnitude—93,000 annually. See *Mortality and Morbidity Weekly Report* 36, no. 42 (October 30, 1987), pp. 693–697.

20. In 1991 these scientists raised the smoking lung cancer death total to 117,000 annually for 1991. See Shepard, Eyre, and Pechacek (1991), and the *New York Times*, August 22, 1991, p. A18.

21. The proportion of smokers age 18 and over in 1985 was 32.7 percent (male) and 27.5 percent (female); in 1965 the proportion of smokers age 18 and over was 53.4 percent (male) and 34.1 percent (female). See the U.S. Department of Health and Human Services (1989), p. 132. The total population of males and females was 88.405 million

(males) and 91.886 million (females) in 1985; and 62.029 (males) and 64.114 million (females) in 1965. See U.S. Department of Commerce (1966, 1985). Combining these sets of statistics enables one to calculate the total number of smokers in 1965 (53.4 million) and 1985 (52.9 million).

22. Ibid.

23. The discussion below draws on the following data. The total death risk estimate of 300,000 deaths per year is from the U.S. Department of Health and Human Services (1988), p. iii. The lung cancer risk estimates were discussed in nn. 19 and 20. This mortality estimate was updated in the subsequent year by the U.S. Department of Health and Human Services (1989), to an estimated smoking-related mortality of 337,000 deaths (p. 22). In addition, the total attributable deaths in 1985 was 390,000, where this figure included "deaths among newborns and infants from maternal smoking, deaths from cigarette-caused residential fires, and lung cancer deaths among nonsmokers due to environmental tobacco smoke" (pp. 22, 160). More recent evidence not yet included in a report by the Surgeon General suggests that the total smoking death toll may have been as high as 434,000 in 1988. See the *New York Times*, February 1, 1991, p. A9.

24. See Combs and Slovic (1979), and Fischhoff et al. (1981).

25. If we let X_{ji} be a vector of variables characterizing each source j of information for person i (i.e., j = 1 for prior beliefs, j = 2 for smoking-related experience, and j = 3 for direct information transfer), and let α_j be the associated vector of coefficients, then the lung cancer risk perception equation to be estimated for person i can be written

$$RISK_i = \alpha_0 + \alpha_1 X_{1i} + \alpha_2 X_{2i} + \alpha_3 X_{3i} + u_i,$$

where u_i is a random error term.

26. In particular, estimates using $\ln(1+RISK)$ yielded almost identical results.

27. These variables represent different X_3 values in the equation.

28. This smoking history 0–1 dummy variable captures the smoking experience variable given by X_2 in equation 2 of the original model.

29. Using the demographic variables and a set of fifty refined regional variables as instruments, one can calculate the instrumental variables estimate for PAST OR CURRENT SMOKER, which is included in addition to the variables included in Table 4–5. This constructed variable had an estimated value of 0.0316 and a standard error of 0.0929, so that one cannot reject the hypothesis that the original PAST OR CURRENT SMOKER variables are not endogenous. The smoking variable consequently passes the Hausman (1978) specification test. The excluded instrument set (i.e., the regional variables) also passes a test of overidentifying restrictions.

30. As indicated in Overholt, Neptune, and Ashraf (1975), 95 percent of all untreated cancer patients die within a year after diagnosis. In contrast, the 1978 American Cancer Society survey found that 71 percent of smokers believed that there is a "very good chance" or a "fairly good chance" that lung cancer could be cured if it is detected early. The quantitative significance of the responses is unclear, and the probability and meaning of early detection are not indicated. The same survey found that smoking led the list of cancer causes in the view of smokers and nonsmokers. See "Public Attitudes toward Cancer and Cancer Tests," *CA-A Cancer Journal for Clinicians* 30 (1980), pp. 92–98.

31. For example, analysis of valuations of nonfatal and fatal forms of lymph cancer by Magat, Viscusi, and Huber (1991) found that curable lymph cancer was equivalent to a lottery involving a .625 probability of death and a .375 probability of good health. Even nonfatal cases of cancer are unattractive prospects.

32. Recall that the mortality risk to the individual of smoking is .18 to .36.

33. U.S. Department of Health, Education, and Welfare (1968). This estimate is cited

in the 1989 Report of the Surgeon General (p. 8), which updates the mortality risk assessments in Chapter 3 but not the loss in life expectancy. See the U.S. Department of Health and Human Services (1989).

34. U.S. Department of Health and Human Services (1989), p. 11.

35. The survey coding of the responses is a bit broad, as the survey does not elicit an estimated life years lost but rather a range: less than 2 years, 2 to 4 years, 6 to 8 years, 8 to 10 years, more than 10 years, and don't know. Coding the individuals who responded more than 10 years is most problematic. I am grateful to Pauline Ippolito for providing me with the text of the original survey.

36. The original reporting of these results is in Viscusi (1988).

37. Using the data from Table 4–11, the overall assessed risk value is .44(.427)1 pack of cigarettes + .35(.225)5 packs of cigarettes = .582 packs of cigarettes.

38. In my food cancer warning study (see Viscusi [1988]), individuals' responses to different risk questions indicated an assessed cancer death risk of 0.21 per pack of cigarettes smoked per day, which led to an implied death risk of 0.33 using 1980 data on the number of cigarettes smoked from data given by the Tobacco Institute (1987), p. 6. Information on the number of smokers appears in the U.S. Department of Commerce (1985), p. 119.

5

The Effect of Risks
on Smoking Behavior

Risk perceptions are only one component of the smoking decision process. The second class of issues pertains to the linkage between risk perceptions and smoking behavior. If risk perceptions did not affect smoking in a significant manner, then doubt would be cast on the rationality of these consumption decisions. In the case of lung cancer risks, smoking behavior is very responsive to risk perceptions in the expected direction.

This analysis of smoking behavior serves as a more general study of the character of risk-taking behavior. Much of the economic literature dealing with consumer and worker responses to risk is based on an assumption of rational individual responses to risk. Although evidence of rationality has been manifested in diverse ways by, for example, individuals' safety-precaution responses involving use of seat belts[1] and the positive effect of job risks on wage rates,[2] these studies almost invariably have not focused on the components of the individuals' decision-making process.[3] In particular, what is the person's market response based on his or her subjective assessment of the risk? Analysts seldom have the detailed information needed to address this issue. This cigarette smoking analysis provides a more refined exploration of this fundamental aspect of behavior than has appeared in any other context.

The character of the data requires the analysis to focus on static consumption decisions. What are individuals' risk perceptions and tastes, and how do these affect observed smoking behavior? The nature of the data analyzed consequently does not permit consideration of changes in smoking behavior, such as decisions to quit smoking. The costs associated with changes in smoking behavior have been recently designated a problem of "addiction" by the Surgeon General.[4] Some recent economic contributions suggest that our interpretation of addiction phenomena is quite complex. There is, for example, a debate among economists over the degree to which addictive behavior is rational.[5] To the extent that costs of change are relevant from the standpoint of market failure, it will be because individuals made mistaken decisions that they wish to reverse.[6]

My analysis will shed light on how smoking behavior would change if risk perceptions were accurate, thus dealing indirectly with some of the factors that affect our assessment of the addiction issue. In effect, the study here can be viewed as the cigarette smoking analogue of the wage equation estimates in the job risk literature. Even though there are transactions costs to job changing, economists have obtained substantial insight from analyzing wage equations and other cross-sectional aspects of labor market behavior.

SMOKING ATTITUDES AND SOURCES OF RISK INFORMATION

The Audits & Surveys study began with an open-ended memory probe regarding individuals' reactions to cigarettes. This innovative technique of eliciting consumer attitudes toward a product in an open-ended manner provides detailed information regarding individuals' assessments of the properties of a product. Although this product reaction measure is not the same as the smoking decision variable, it is an excellent measure of the attractiveness of the product, as it will affect consumer behavior. In addition, by placing this question at the start of a survey, one is able to obtain responses that are not tainted by subsequent questions that might, for example, highlight the importance of the product's risks as a salient product attribute.

Table 5–1 summarizes the survey responses listed in order of decreasing frequency. For each of these reactions (e.g., causes lung cancer), Table 5–1 gives the fraction of the individuals in each of the smoking groups who made that particular statement in the open-ended memory recall (REACTION). Table 5–1 also includes the mean lung cancer risk assessment (RISK) corresponding to that group. What is most stunning is the overwhelmingly adverse sentiment against the product, even among current product users. Individuals cite risks of lung cancer, general causes of cancer, and annoyance from cigarette smoke. The diversity of the adverse reactions to cigarettes is quite striking and is possibly unequaled by any other widely used consumer product.

Consider the most prominent responses listed in Table 5–1. Almost half of the sample indicated that cigarette smoking was annoying or mentioned some other adverse effect of cigarettes not related to health. One-third of the sample indicated that cigarettes cause disease, and over one-fifth of the respondents indicated that cigarette smoking causes cancer in general. This cancer response is in addition to the 15 percent of the sample that indicated that cigarettes cause lung cancer. Similarly, one-fifth of the sample indicated that cigarette smoking was polluting, or they mentioned other health effects. Even some of the less prominent responses reflect a variety of health concerns pertaining to the shortening of life or knowledge of people who have experienced these adverse health effects because of smoking. By almost any standard, there is a very strong negative reaction to cigarettes in terms of the character of the initial responses that individuals have to this product.

The only apparently positive responses are the 12 percent of respondents, all of whom are smokers, who gave reasons for smoking; the 2.1 percent of the respondents who indicate that hearing about cigarettes makes them want one; the 1.3 percent of the population who were skeptical of the warnings and did not believe that smoking is harmful; and the fewer than 1 percent of the respondents who indicate that hearing about cigarettes reminds them of the product advertising.

Table 5–1   Distribution of responses to open-ended memory probe

Reaction to cigarette mention	Fraction with reaction (REACTION) and their risk perception (RISK)							
	Full sample		Current smoker		Former smoker		Nonsmoker	
	Reaction	Risk	Reaction	Risk	Reaction	Risk	Reaction	Risk
Annoying, non–health-related effects	.420	.457	.157	.396	.424	.419	.550	.481
Causes other disease, affects health	.328	.444	.185	.392	.385	.424	.371	.468
Causes cancer (general)	.221	.439	.155	.353	.249	.420	.240	.477
Polluting, other health-related effects	.200	.453	.053	.362	.195	.399	.276	.481
Causes lung cancer	.151	.436	.092	.342	.145	.445	.184	.457
Expensive, costly	.130	.428	.125	.343	.149	.408	.123	.482
Reasons for smoking (all mentions)	.117	.364	.424	.358	.030	.386	.007	.482
Have quit/used to smoke	.096	.393	.003	.100	.370	.394	.006	.402
Bad, dangerous to health (general)	.073	.437	.076	.373	.066	.438	.075	.468
Shortens life, kills	.071	.469	.032	.446	.083	.440	.084	.488
Know people who died or got diseases because of smoking	.065	.455	.023	.393	.072	.485	.083	.451
Trying/have tried to quit	.058	.394	.228	.393	.004	.443	—	—
Public has been made aware of dangers to health	.056	.385	.059	.325	.058	.409	.053	.405
People should be allowed to make own choice	.033	.337	.036	.279	.034	.337	.031	.372
More should be done to discourage smoking	.027	.478	.013	.470	.036	.440	.029	.503
Hazardous, not health-related	.022	.433	.009	.381	.032	.382	.023	.478
Hearing of cigarettes makes me want one	.021	.380	.077	.375	.008	.425	—	—
Never want to smoke	.019	.429	—	—	.012	.298	.033	.452
Smokers are crazy, idiots	.017	.529	.012	.260	.017	.558	.020	.592
Skeptical, don't believe smoking harmful	.013	.266	.044	.235	.006	.234	.002	.667
Don't like smoking/people shouldn't smoke (general)	.013	.357	.004	.500	.013	.356	.017	.342
Causes other types of cancer	.009	.408	.005	.475	.013	.391	.010	.401

The reaction of smokers to a mention of cigarettes is also quite interesting. One would have expected almost all individuals who currently purchase a product to be enthusiastic about it. What we find instead is that there are a large number of negative mentions of cigarettes from the smoking population. Although two-fifths of all the smokers give some reason for smoking as their initial reaction to the memory recall task, 16 percent of the sample mentioned annoying nonhealth effects, 19 percent of all smokers mentioned causes of disease, 16 percent mentioned causes of general cancer, and 9 percent mentioned that smoking causes lung cancer. Many of the other less prominent mentions are also quite negative in character as, for example, 23 percent of the sample's first reaction is that they have tried to quit and 8 percent indicate that smoking is bad and dangerous to one's health.

The patterns of risk perception associated with reactions are surprisingly similar. The highest risk assessment comes from the group who responded "smokers are crazy, idiots"; this group of respondents had an average risk perception of .53. At the lowest end in terms of the risk assessment were individuals who are "skeptical, don't believe smoking harmful," who had an average risk assessment of .27. This perception is lower than the sample average but is nevertheless much greater than the "true" risk level.

Similar patterns are borne out by the individual responses for the smoking groups as well. However, with narrowly defined groups, often there is a small sample problem. If we only examine the cigarette mentions that occurred in at least 1 percent of the cases for the sample, for cigarette smokers the lowest risk assessment is .26, and this is for the category of individuals who smoke but who claim that "smokers are crazy, idiots." Somewhat surprisingly, perhaps because of the very small number of observations in this cell, we get the opposite pattern that we find in the full sample, where individuals with this response have the highest risk assessment.

Specific mentions of public health warnings do not appear to make a substantial difference in the responses. The sample participants who indicate that the public has been made aware of the dangers of smoking to one's health have a risk assessment that averages .39 for the entire sample and is not too dissimilar from that for society at large.

Perhaps the most interesting category from the standpoint of smoking behavior consists of individuals who gave "reasons for smoking" (all mentions). Over 40 percent of current smokers fell into this group, and for this group of current smokers who have prosmoking attitudes, the perceived risk assessment is .36. Moreover, even for the current smokers who said that they were "skeptical, don't believe smoking is harmful," the perceived risk assessment is .24. For individuals with a wide variety of smoking attitudes, there is evidence of substantial risk perception.

There does not appear to be any systematic pattern in which there are major risk-information gaps among the population segments. There are no obvious population groups who have failed to obtain information about the potential hazards of cigarette smoking.

An additional perspective on the nature of individual reactions to cigarettes is obtained by analyzing how these reactions vary with respect to the different information the individual may have heard about smoking behavior. The columns in Table 5–2 provide each of the eight possible informational outcomes, in particular whether or not the individuals have heard particular statements about smoking. For example, the first column of statistics provides the memory recall reactions to cigarette smoking for the portion of the sample that has heard that smoking shortens life, whereas the second column of statistics pertains to the fraction of the sample who have not heard that smoking shortens life. Below each of the risk-perception numbers is the fraction of the individuals in the particular cell who fall into that class. Thus, 60.2 percent of those individuals who have heard smoking shortens life also indicate that smoking causes lung cancer, and these people have a risk perception of .45. For the individuals in the sample who have not heard that smoking shortens life, 39.8 percent believe that smoking causes lung cancer, and this group of respondents assesses the lung cancer risk posed by cigarettes as being .42.

Because of the refined nature of the divisions provided by this table, the sample sizes in many of the cells are relatively small, particularly compared with many of the previous tables that have been examined. In part as a result of this limited sample size, we observe greater variations in the table since outliers play a more significant role.

Overall, there seem to be no major differences across the different kinds of reactions to cigarettes in terms of the information that the subjects have acquired. For the twenty-four different memory probe responses to cigarettes that appear in Table 5–2, the fraction of individuals who have heard that smoking shortens life ranges from .50 to .73. For the information "have heard smoking is dangerous to health" the range is from .64 to .81. The fraction of people who have heard "smoking is bad for health but not dangerous" ranges from .53 to .72. Finally, the fraction who indicated that they "have heard smoking is not bad for health" ranges from .43 to .72.

What is particularly striking is that for every one of the 192 different possible combinations of information that people have heard about cigarettes and stated reactions to cigarettes, the risk perception greatly exceeds scientists' estimates of the actual lung cancer risk of cigarette smoking. Consider some of the risk responses for several of the key attitudinal responses. For the response that smoking "causes lung cancer" the risk assessment range is from .42 to .46. This pattern is also borne out by other negative mentions of cigarettes.

The positive mentions of cigarettes are associated with lower risk-perception levels, but the variation within these groups does not appear to be substantial. For people who are "skeptical, don't believe smoking is harmful," the risk-perception range goes from .23 for individuals who "have heard smoking shortens life" to .31 for people who "have not heard smoking is bad for health but not dangerous." What is most striking about this final set of responses is that for people who are skeptical about smoking risks and do not believe that smoking is harmful, the information that they may have heard does not seem to have made

Table 5–2 Risk perceptions based on information and the attitudes toward cigarettes

Cigarette mention	Conditional fraction in cell (average RISK perception)							
	Have heard smoking shortens life	Have not heard smoking shortens life	Have heard smoking is dangerous to health	Have not heard smoking is dangerous to health	Have heard smoking is bad for health but not dangerous	Have not heard smoking is bad for health but not dangerous	Have heard smoking is not bad for health	Have not heard smoking is not bad for health
Causes lung cancer	.602 (.445)	.398 (.424)	.708 (.444)	.292 (.417)	.617 (.423)	.383 (.458)	.572 (.427)	.428 (.449)
Causes other types of cancer	.655 (.409)	.345 (.405)	.690 (.419)	.310 (.383)	.655 (.413)	.345 (.398)	.724 (.377)	.276 (.490)
Causes cancer (general)	.630 (.438)	.370 (.442)	.698 (.431)	.302 (.458)	.665 (.438)	.335 (.443)	.570 (.441)	.430 (.438)
Shortens life, kills	.700 (.467)	.300 (.473)	.727 (.463)	.273 (.487)	.591 (.455)	.409 (.490)	.559 (.485)	.441 (.449)
Causes other diseases, effects	.640 (.443)	.360 (.447)	.714 (.439)	.286 (.459)	.636 (.437)	.364 (.458)	.573 (.455)	.427 (.431)
Addictive, habit-forming, like a drug	.609 (.414)	.391 (.430)	.676 (.404)	.324 (.456)	.668 (.426)	.332 (.409)	.567 (.430)	.433 (.408)
Know people who died or got diseases because of smoking	.725 (.447)	.275 (.477)	.750 (.454)	.250 (.459)	.583 (.463)	.417 (.445)	.510 (.472)	.490 (.438)

Polluting, other health-related effects	.667 (.450)	.333 (.459)	.720 (.457)	.280 (.442)	.595 (.452)	.405 (.455)	.545 (.461)	.455 (.444)
Bad, dangerous to health (general)	.656 (.403)	.344 (.501)	.678 (.409)	.322 (.496)	.599 (.442)	.401 (.429)	.559 (.439)	.441 (.433)
Expensive, costly	.589 (.425)	.411 (.431)	.678 (.412)	.322 (.460)	.658 (.421)	.342 (.440)	.599 (.435)	.401 (.416)
Smokers are crazy, idiots	.630 (.473)	.370 (.623)	.648 (.504)	.352 (.573)	.611 (.559)	.389 (.481)	.611 (.561)	.389 (.477)
Trying, have tried to quit	.591 (.394)	.409 (.394)	.635 (.385)	.365 (.410)	.619 (.393)	.381 (.396)	.597 (.395)	.403 (.392)
Have quit, used to smoke	.634 (.383)	.366 (.410)	.695 (.389)	.305 (.401)	.658 (.390)	.342 (.397)	.587 (.410)	.413 (.367)
Having cigarettes makes me want one	.652 (.356)	.348 (.423)	.667 (.375)	.333 (.390)	.561 (.369)	.439 (.393)	.576 (.376)	.424 (.384)
Never want to smoke	.700 (.420)	.300 (.451)	.650 (.422)	.350 (.442)	.683 (.440)	.317 (.406)	.600 (.451)	.400 (.396)
Public has been made aware of dangers to health	.626 (.381)	.374 (.391)	.701 (.386)	.299 (.383)	.655 (.376)	.345 (.402)	.586 (.402)	.414 (.360)
More should be done to discourage smoking	.578 (.463)	.422 (.498)	.639 (.476)	.361 (.481)	.723 (.469)	.277 (.502)	.675 (.456)	.325 (.522)
People should be allowed to make own choice	.716 (.353)	.284 (.297)	.814 (.343)	.186 (.312)	.559 (.331)	.441 (.346)	.431 (.366)	.569 (.316)

(continued)

Table 5–2 (*Continued*)

Cigarette mention	Conditional fraction in cell (average RISK perception)							
	Have heard smoking shortens life	Have not heard smoking shortens life	Have heard smoking is dangerous to health	Have not heard smoking is dangerous to health	Have heard smoking is bad for health but not dangerous	Have not heard smoking is bad for health but not dangerous	Have heard smoking is not bad for health	Have not heard smoking is not bad for health
Annoying, non–health-related effects	.638 (.447)	.362 (.477)	.688 (.452)	.312 (.469)	.614 (.454)	.386 (.463)	.578 (.460)	.422 (.453)
Reasons for smoking (all mentions)	.597 (.380)	.403 (.340)	.677 (.375)	.323 (.340)	.660 (.336)	.340 (.417)	.567 (.340)	.433 (.395)
Skeptical, don't believe smoking harmful	.500 (.232)	.500 (.299)	.738 (.275)	.262 (.239)	.690 (.247)	.310 (.308)	.548 (.292)	.452 (.234)
Hazardous, not health-related	.676 (.423)	.324 (.454)	.735 (.404)	.265 (.513)	.647 (.448)	.353 (.405)	.632 (.461)	.368 (.385)
Makes me think of advertising	.556 (.368)	.444 (.340)	.778 (.413)	.222 (.155)	.722 (.378)	.278 (.296)	.556 (.342)	.444 (.373)
Don't like smoking, people shouldn't smoke (general)	.675 (.361)	.325 (.350)	.700 (.356)	.300 (.360)	.525 (.383)	.475 (.328)	.500 (.354)	.500 (.361)

much difference in influencing their risk assessments. In some instances having heard adverse information raises the risk assessment, whereas in other cases it seems to lower their risk assessment.

The response category that is second most favorable toward cigarettes also does not reflect any obviously apparent informational inadequacy. This group of individuals are those who believe "people should be allowed to make own choice." Individuals who have heard that smoking shortens life and who have this reaction to cigarettes have a higher risk assessment than those who have not heard that smoking shortens life. However, people who have heard that smoking is not bad for their health have a higher risk assessment than do people who have *not* heard that smoking is not bad for their health. The role of the informational background has inconsistent effects, as no clear pattern emerges. This lack of a consistent or predictable pattern suggests that these various statements about smoking do not have strong informational content given respondents' other knowledge of the risks of smoking.

Perhaps the main implication of this refined breakdown of information about knowledge about smoking risks, risk perceptions, and reactions to cigarettes is that for every segment of the population that can be isolated there is evidence of substantial risk assessments. Moreover, there are no major differences in the responses depending on what particular informational group the individual may be in. These results are quite consistent with individuals having a well-developed concept of the risks of smoking that will not be significantly affected by particular pieces of knowledge they may or may not have heard.

There does, however, appear to be a much stronger relationship between the informational questions and the overall reactions to cigarettes. Comparison of the informational knowledge questions based on the smoking attitude response suggests fairly similar knowledge responses across smoking attitudes. Roughly two-thirds of the individuals in all of the smoking reaction categories have heard either that smoking shortens life or that smoking is dangerous to health. Similarly, roughly an equal fraction of the sample has heard that smoking is bad for health but not dangerous. The fraction of the sample that has heard that smoking is not bad for health is consistently somewhat less but nevertheless in the vicinity of three-fifths, and once again there do not appear to be substantial differences in this fraction across the different memory recall response groups.

THE SMOKING PROBABILITY EQUATION

The presence of substantial risk perceptions and adverse reactions to cigarettes does not necessarily imply that individuals will be making sound decisions with respect to cigarette smoking. What we must then determine is the extent to which there is a linkage of these various factors with the smoking decision. In particular, to what extent is there a responsiveness to cigarette risk perceptions that influences the smoking probability?

Assessing the link between smoking risk perceptions and smoking behavior will address a recurring issue that has arisen in the smoking debate. Smoking critics often charge that even if people are cognizant of the risks, their decisions will still be flawed.[7] First, even if they understand the risks to smokers at large, they may not believe that their own risk is that great. Second, smokers may try to selectively ignore adverse information about an activity that they find attractive.

These stylized views certainly are not consistent with the adverse reactions that respondents expressed regarding cigarettes. Even smokers do not idealize the attributes of this product and have a predominantly negative view of many of the product's consequences. The extent to which these adverse product assessments are borne out in smoking behavior will also prove to be quite powerful.

Table 5–3 presents five alternative specifications that represent different operationalizations of a model of the determinants of the probability that an individual smokes.[8] To recognize the constrained nature of the smoking probability (it cannot exceed 1 or be below 0), a logit estimation procedure is employed. Each equation includes a series of seven regional dummy variables to capture regional differences in prices and tastes for cigarettes. Equation 1 in Table 5–3 includes the basic set of demographic variables to capture smoking tastes and a RISK variable to capture smoking losses. Chapter 6 will explore age interactions with RISK as well as a model in which smoking decisions and risk perceptions are part of a simultaneous equations system.

As expected, higher perceived risks of significant cigarette smoking reduce the smoking probability, as RISK has a negative effect. Although the RISK variable could potentially be endogenous, with smoking behavior influencing risk beliefs this possibility is explored and rejected.[9] Nevertheless, Chapter 6 will report results that control for this complication as well. The principal taste variables of consequence are for AGE22–45 and MALE smokers, each of which has a higher smoking propensity than average.

The second equation adds the set of four informational variables to capture aspects of risk perceptions not fully captured by RISK. Individuals who have heard that smoking reduces one's life expectancy (SHORTENS LIFE) are less likely to smoke, and somewhat surprisingly a similar effect is observed for those who have heard that smoking is not bad for one's health (NOT BAD FOR HEALTH). Since such statements include little information that is new, the ideas heard variables probably capture in part omitted influences correlated with these variables. This interpretation is consistent with the results for equations 4 and 5 in Table 5–3, where the addition of the attitude probe variables strengthens the expected negative effect of SHORTENS LIFE and leads the surprisingly negative role of NOT BAD FOR HEALTH to be statistically insignificant.

The last three equations report results with the attitude probe variables added, where equation 3 excludes the set of Ideas Heard variables and equation 5 omits RISK. The attitude probe variable set captures both taste-related factors and factors related to risk perceptions. All of the attitude probe variables that are significant in any of equations 3 through 5 are significant in all three equations. The negative attitude probe questions that are statistically significant have a negative sign except for the following: HABIT-FORMING, TRIED TO QUIT, and HEARING MAKES WANT. Although these are not favorable reactions to cigarettes, the statements are most likely to have been made by smokers who are

Table 5–3 Smoking probability equations, logit model

Independent variables	Coefficients (asymptotic standard errors)				
	1	2	3	4	5
Intercept	−0.9788[a]	−0.5472[a]	−0.7645[a]	−0.3101[a]	−0.7281[a]
	(0.1679)	(0.2283)	(0.2758)	(0.3629)	(0.3431)
RISK	−1.0817[a]	−1.0965[a]	−0.7991[a]	−0.9152[a]	—
	(0.1645)	(0.1652)	(0.2231)	(0.2513)	
AGE16–21	−0.2396	−0.2872	−0.0373	−0.0873	−0.1611
	(0.1663)	(0.1671)	(0.2435)	(0.2451)	(0.2439)
AGE22–45	0.4222[a]	0.3936[a]	0.6480[a]	0.6273[a]	0.6212[a]
	(0.0925)	(0.0923)	(0.1489)	(0.1501)	(0.1494)
MALE	0.1253[a]	0.1329[a]	0.0572	0.0672	0.1159
	(0.0874)	(0.0876)	(0.1339)	(0.1343)	(0.1333)
HOUSEHOLD SIZE	0.0010	0.0020	−0.0722	−0.0711	−0.0764
	(0.0230)	(0.0453)	(0.0701)	(0.0702)	(0.0700)
Ideas heard					
SHORTENS LIFE	—	−0.2678[a]	—	−0.3812[a]	−0.3836[a]
		(0.1198)		(0.1811)	(0.1814)
DANGEROUS TO HEALTH	—	−0.1385	—	−0.0579	−0.0181
		(0.1230)		(0.1890)	(0.1882)
BAD, NOT DANGEROUS	—	−0.0007	—	−0.0343	−0.0147
		(0.1207)		(0.1834)	(0.1830)
NOT BAD FOR HEALTH	—	−0.2795[a]	—	−0.2640	−0.2512
		(0.1196)		(0.1826)	(0.1827)
Attitude probe—negative					
CAUSES LUNG CANCER	—	—	−0.4790[a]	−0.5122[a]	−0.5110[a]
			(0.2059)	(0.2073)	(0.2059)
CAUSES OTHER CANCER	—	—	−0.1217	−0.0344	−0.1056
			(0.8391)	(0.8354)	(0.8392)
CAUSES ANY CANCER	—	—	−0.3909[a]	−0.3901[a]	−0.4000[a]
			(0.1664)	(0.1667)	(0.1659)
SHORTENS LIFE	—	—	−0.1802	−0.1545	−0.1867
			(0.3184)	(0.3192)	(0.3195)
AFFECTS HEALTH	—	—	−0.7033[a]	−0.7028[a]	−0.7112[a]
			(0.1620)	(0.1624)	(0.1615)
HABIT-FORMING	—	—	0.4839[a]	0.4734[a]	0.4687[a]
			(0.1934)	(0.1939)	(0.1941)
KNOW PEOPLE DIED	—	—	−1.0068[a]	−0.9851[a]	−1.0042[a]
			(0.4271)	(0.4274)	(0.4255)
POLLUTION EFFECTS	—	—	−1.1864[a]	−1.1953[a]	−1.2006[a]
			(0.2243)	(0.2244)	(0.2541)
GENERAL HEALTH EFFECTS	—	—	−0.4404[a]	−0.4433[a]	−0.4974[a]
			(0.2552)	(0.2559)	(0.2541)

(*continued*)

Table 5–3   (*Continued*)

Independent variables	Coefficients (asymptotic standard errors)				
	1	2	3	4	5
SMOKING EXPENSIVE	—	—	−0.0842 (0.2069)	−0.0768 (0.2071)	−0.0676 (0.2055)
SMOKING STUPID	—	—	−0.5921 (0.6528)	−0.5885 (0.6485)	−0.6801 (0.6332)
TRIED TO QUIT	—	—	5.8869[a] (0.6287)	5.9120[a] (0.6317)	5.9573[a] (0.6381)
USED TO SMOKE	—	—	−4.8643[a] (0.8701)	−4.8676[a] (0.8736)	−4.8338[a] (0.8874)
HEARING MAKES WANT	—	—	3.1760[a] (0.5692)	3.1960[a] (0.5671)	3.1952[a] (0.5653)
NEVER WANT TO	—	—	−9.8398 (52.77)	−9.8257 (52.57)	−9.8031 (52.77)
AWARE OF WARNINGS	—	—	−0.1909 (0.3009)	−0.1971 (0.2995)	−0.1716 (0.2976)
ABOLISH ADS	—	—	−0.3600 (0.5157)	−0.3776 (0.5188)	−0.4244 (0.5141)
FREE CHOICE TO DIE	—	—	−0.1129 (0.3309)	−0.1019 (0.3336)	−0.0395 (0.3196)
NEGATIVE NONHEALTH EFFECTS	—	—	−1.6616[a] (0.1604)	−1.6625[a] (0.1612)	−1.6818[a] (0.1603)
PEOPLE SHOULDN'T	—	—	−2.3596[a] (0.7400)	−2.3985[a] (0.7429)	−2.3891[a] (0.7557)
Attitude probe—positive					
REASONS FOR SMOKING	—	—	3.7010[a] (0.2456)	3.7118[a] (0.2470)	3.7392[a] (0.2458)
DOESN'T BELIEVE WARNINGS	—	—	2.4493[a] (0.6153)	2.4122[a] (0.6206)	2.4889[a] (0.6304)
NONHEALTH HAZARDS	—	—	−0.7987 (0.6819)	−0.7771 (0.6863)	−0.7391 (0.6687)
RECALL ADS	—	—	−4.4038[a] (1.530)	−4.3201[a] (1.575)	−4.3215[a] (1.6160)
Log likelihood	−1699.4	−1693.4	−818.5	−815.13	−821.93

[a] Denotes coefficients that are statistically significant at the 5 percent level, one-tailed test.

not entirely happy with their smoking behavior. If this is the case, these responses will be positively correlated with the dependent variable—being a
smoker at the present time.

   Two positive attitude mentions—REASONS FOR SMOKING and DOESN'T
BELIEVE WARNINGS—raise the smoking probability, controlling for RISK
and other factors, as expected. The individuals whose first reaction to cigarettes

Table 5–4 Summary of instrumental variable estimate of risk variable in the smoking equation

	Equation specification			
	1	2	3	4
RISK (instrumental variables) coefficient (standard error)	−1.0642 (0.1897)	−1.0754 (0.1897)	−0.9189 (0.2926)	−0.9385 (0.2941)
Variables included	Demographics	Demographics ideas heard	Demographics attitude probe	Demographics ideas heard attitude probe

is that they made them RECALL ADS for smoking are less likely to smoke, so that prominence of cigarette advertising in one's memory does not lead to a higher smoking propensity.

The smoking probability equation is based on an assumption that the smoking risk will be captured by the lung cancer risk variable RISK. Although these measures are likely to be strongly correlated, in general RISK will not equal the total assessed smoking risk. The practice of estimating behavioral responses to risk using a single risk variable is a standard practice in literature, as exemplified by studies of compensating wage differentials for job risk, which generally focus on accident fatalities.[10] Nevertheless, there may be a resulting bias in coefficients arising from the types of risk other than lung cancer.[11] The instrumental variables results in Table 5–4 provide efficient estimates of the RISK variable that address this bias problem, and they differ very little from the estimates in Table 5–3, suggesting that the extent of any bias in the results may not be great.

THE EFFECT OF UNBIASED PERCEPTIONS

A principal policy and welfare issue is what effect accurate risk perceptions would have on smoking behavior. If individuals who underestimated the risk or overestimated the risk had a more accurate risk perception and acted upon it, what effect would there be on smoking behavior? Although the data do not make it possible to undertake such an assessment for all smoking risks, we can analyze how responsive smoking decisions would be to different lung cancer risk assessments. This exercise will also be instructive in indicating how responsive smoking behavior is to changes in the lung cancer risk assessment.

Using the results in Table 5–3 (equation 1), one can undertake such calculations by replacing the individual's actual risk perceptions with an estimate of the true risk. Because of the nonlinearity of the logit estimation procedure, the approach here will not be to examine the effects at the variable mean but rather will be a complete simulation for each case. For each of the 3,119 sample members I calculate the predicted smoking probability based on their reported risk perceptions and the predicted probability with accurate risk perceptions. These calculations were undertaken for two true lung cancer risk levels—.05 and .10.

Table 5—5   Effect of lung cancer risk-perception biases on smoking probability

	True lung cancer risk = .05		True lung cancer risk = .10	
	Underassess risk, RISK < .05	Do not underassess risk, RISK ≥ .05	Underassess risk, RISK < .10	Do not underassess risk, RISK ≥ .10
Fraction of sample	.052	.948	.097	.903
Current smoking probability	.337	.245	.329	.241
Smoking probability, if accurate perceptions (i.e., RISK = .05)	.328	.327		
Smoking probability, if accurate perceptions (i.e., RISK = .10)			.313	.315
Change in smoking probability	−.009	+0.082	−.016	+.074

Table 5–5 summarizes the results of these calculations. Consider first the results for the true lung cancer risk = .05 case. For individuals who underassess the risk, they do so by very little, so that accurate risk perceptions would diminish their smoking probability by .009, or under 1 percent. For individuals who do not underassess the risk, the smoking probability would increase substantially—by .082—if risk perceptions were unbiased.

To ascertain the overall effect on societal smoking rates, these estimates must be weighted by the fraction of individuals in the group. Since many more individuals overassess or correctly assess the risk rather than underassess the risk (.948 versus .052), the societal effect is driven almost entirely by the influence of those who do not underassess the risk. Overall, accurate lung cancer risk perceptions would boost the societal smoking rate by 7.5 percent. Smoking rates would increase by roughly one-fourth of their current levels if people believed that the true lung cancer risk was .05.

These results are not particularly sensitive to increases in the true lung cancer risk level that is assumed since overassessments of the risk are of greater magnitude. For the true risk value of .10, the decreased smoking probability for the risk underassessors is almost double that of before, but the population share with this response remains small. The decreased smoking probability of those who do not underassess the risk has dropped somewhat, and a change of equal consequence is that the fraction of individuals in this group has dropped as well. The net effect is that the societal smoking rate would rise by 6.5 percent if individuals believed the risk level was .10.

The role of risk underestimation for lung cancer risks is dwarfed by the effect of risk overestimation. An unbiased assessment of this component of smoking risks based on current scientific evidence would boost cigarette smoking because of the skewed distribution of risk perceptions around the true lung cancer risk level.

CIGARETTE DEMAND AND THE LUNG CANCER RISK
EQUIVALENT OF EXCISE TAXES

Although risk perceptions clearly will influence the demand for cigarettes nega-
tively, other factors also affect consumer demand for products. Chief among
these is the price of the product, which is affected not only by the production
costs associated with cigarettes but also by the specific taxes imposed on cigarettes. The effect of each of these will be influenced by the elasticity of consumer
demand with respect to the cigarette price.

If we take the extreme case of cigarette addiction as a reference point, current
cigarette smokers will have no responsiveness whatsoever to the price of cigarettes if they are completely locked into their current consumption behavior.
Similarly, if one hypothesizes a model in which cigarette smoking decisions are
driven completely by concerns other than economics, the demand for cigarette
products will not be altered by changes in the price. Even addictive drugs, such
as heroin, exhibit price responsiveness so that the existence of some price elasticity does not rule out all addictive properties. Moreover, models of "rational
addiction," such as those formulated by Becker and Murphy (1988), explicitly
allow for price sensitivity.

An extensive set of studies of cigarette smoking demand indicates quite consistently that the nature of consumers' demand for cigarettes is not entirely
dissimilar from their demand for other products. Table 5–6 summarizes the
implications of forty-one studies that have examined the price and income elasticities (i.e., percentage change in cigarette demand in response to a percentage
change in price or income) of cigarette demand. The variation in consumer
demand for cigarettes with respect to income is ambiguous from a theoretical
standpoint. Cigarette consumption could be a normal good for which the level of
consumer demand increases with income. Alternatively, it could also be an
inferior good for which consumer demand drops with income levels. In either
case, the presence of such behavior gives us no guidance whatsoever with respect
to the extent to which these decisions are rational.

The studies in Table 5–6 generally indicate that cigarette consumption is a
normal good that increases with income but less than proportionally. Although
some of the elasticity estimates fall outside of the range [0,1], most of the income
elasticity estimates are clustered in that interval, and only five of the studies
reporting income elasticities have found a negative income elasticity. In each
case of a negative income elasticity, the magnitude of the elasticity was very
close to 0 or the elasticity varied in sign with different years so that the overall
consensus in the literature is that more affluent individuals are likely to purchase
cigarettes.

It should be emphasized that these effects ideally isolate the role of income
status and do not reflect the role of population characteristics correlated with
income. For example, consumer demand might drop with educational level and
rise with total income, but ideally the statistical analyses should distinguish the
specific influence of each of these factors. This is, however, difficult to do using
the aggregative data that have been the focus of most of these studies.

Table 5–6 Empirical studies of the demand for cigarettes

		Estimated elasticities	
Author (date)	Data and source (method)	Price	Income
Schoenberg (1933)	U.S. time series 1923–1931 1913–1931 per capita consumption U.S. Internal Revenue Service (ordinary least squares)	−0.68 −0.25	— —
Gottsegen (1940)	U.S. family budget 1918–1919 U.S. Bureau of Labor Statistics (arc-elasticity)	—	0.81
Tennant (1950)	U.S. time series 1913–1945 per capita consumption U.S. Department of Agriculture (ordinary least squares)	—	0.46
Stone (1954)	U.K. time series 1920–1938 aggregate tobacco consumption (ordinary least squares)	−0.48	−0.13
Maier (1955)	State cross sections 1947–1951 each year estimated separately	−0.38 −0.31 to −1.48	0.60 0.29 to 0.60
Koutsoyannis (1963)	U.S. time series 1950–1959 aggregate tobacco consumption international results	−0.937 −0.036 to −0.951	0.337 0.066 to 0.828
Lyon and Simon (1968)	State tax increases 1951–1964 median arc-elasticity Tobacco Tax Council (quasi-experimental method)	−0.511	
Vernon, Rives, and Naylor (1969)	U.S. time series 1949–1964 (19-equation econometric model of tobacco industry)	−0.43	0.77
Houthakker and Taylor (1970)	U.S. time series 1929–1964 personal consumption expenditures Survey of Current Business U.S. Department of Commerce (three-pass least squares)	−0.456 (short-run) −1.892 (long-run)	
Laughhunn and Lyon (1971)	Pooled state cross section, time series 1950–1968 Tobacco Tax Council (Bayesian regression)	−0.81	0.42
Sumner (1971)	U.K. annual time series 1951– 1967 quarterly 1955:1–1968:2 per capita expenditures (ordinary least squares)	−0.238 −0.134 to −0.831	0.480 0.268 to 0.645
Hamilton (1972)	State cross sections 1954, 1965 each year separately (ordinary least squares)	−0.511	0.734 0.726 to 0.821

(*continued*)

Table 5–6 (Continued)

Author (date)	Data and source (method)	Estimated elasticities	
		Price	Income
Schmalansee (1972)	U.S. time series 1947–1967 per capita consumption industry data (ordinary least squares)	−0.316 (short-run) −1.090 (long-run)	0.323 (short-run) 1.114 (long-run)
Schnabel (1972)	U.S. time series 1949–1963 per capita consumption U.S. Department of Agriculture U.S. Bureau of Labor Statistics (ordinary least squares)	−0.85 (short-run)	0.35 (short-run)
Russell (1973)	U.K. time series 1946–1971 per capita male consumption Tobacco Research Council H. M. Customs and Excises (ordinary least squares)	−0.59 −0.50 to −0.66	
Atkinson and Skegg (1973)	U.K. time series 1951–1970 per capita consumption Tobacco Research Council (ordinary least squares)	−0.115 +0.002 to −0.480	0.626 0.174 to 1.340
Atkinson and Skegg (1974)	U.K. time series 1951–1970 per capita male consumption Russell (1973) Atkinson and Skegg (1973) (ordinary least squares)	−0.01 −0.01 to −0.62	0.36 0.09 to 0.36
Peto (1974)	U.K. time series 1951–1970 per capita male consumption (Cochrane-Orcutt procedure)	−0.37 to −0.64	0.14 to 0.49
McGuinness and Cowling (1975)	U.K. time series 1957:2–1968:4 aggregate expenditures (U.K. Central Statistical Office) (ordinary least squares)	−0.985 (short-run) −1.045 (long-run)	0.311 (short-run) 0.330 (long-run)
Warner (1977)	U.S. time series 1947–1970 per capita consumption U.S. Department of Agriculture	−0.511 (extraneous)	
Ippolito, Murphy, and Sant (1979)	U.S. time series 1926–1975 per capita consumption Federal Trade Commission (Cochrane-Orcutt procedure)	−0.811	0.735
Fujii (1980)	U.S. time series 1929–1973 per capita consumption Hamilton (1972) extended national income accounts (ridge regression)	−0.475 to −0.627 (short-run) −0.708 to −0.929 (long-run)	0.220 to 0.339 (short-run) 0.329 to 0.499 (long-run)
Schneider, Klein, and Murphy (1981)	U.S. time series 1930–1978 per capita consumption U.S. Department of Agriculture U.S. Bureau of Labor Statistics (ordinary least squares)	−1.218 (cigarettes) −0.949 (tobacco)	0.462 (extraneous) 0.462 (tobacco)

(continued)

Table 5–6 (*Continued*)

Author (date)	Data and source (method)	Estimated elasticities	
		Price	Income
Witt and Pass (1981)	U.K. time series 1955–1975 per capita consumption Tobacco Research Council *U.K. Annual Abstract of Statistics State Review of Press and TV Advertising* (ordinary least squares)	−0.321	0.126
Warner (1981)	U.S. time series 1947–1978 per capita consumption U.S. Department of Agriculture (ordinary least squares)	−0.37 (short-run)	
Lewit, Coate, and Grossman (1981)	U.S. micro cross section 1966, 1970 youths age 12–17 years Health Examination Survey U.S. National Center for Health Statistics (ordinary least squares)	−1.44	
Lewit and Coate (1982)	U.S. micro cross section 1976 National Health Interview Survey U.S. National Center for Health Statistics Tobacco Tax Council (ordinary least squares)	−0.416 −0.025 to −1.401	0.080
Witt and Pass (1983)	U.K. time series 1955–1975 Data are the same used by Witt and Pass (1981) (ordinary least squares)	−0.167 to −0.349	0.126 to 0.316
Young (1983)	U.S. time series 1929–1973 Data are the same as used by Fujii (1980) (ridge regression)	−0.334 (short-run)	0.274 (short-run)
Leu (1984)	Switzerland time series 1954–1981 per capita consumption (ordinary least squares)	−1.00	−.93
Sumner and Alston (1984)	U.S. time series 1946–1983 (generalized least squares)	−0.29	0.11
Bishop and Yoo (1985)	U.S. time series 1954–1980 aggregate consumption U.S. Department of Agriculture (three-stage least squares)	−0.454	0.919
Sullivan (1985)	U.S. state panel 1955–1982 Tobacco Tax Council (generalized least squares)	−0.655	
Baltagi and Levin (1986)	U.S. state panel 1963–1980 U.S. Federal Trade Commission (Hausman-Taylor estimation)	−0.215 (short-run)	−0.0002 (short-run)

(*continued*)

Table 5–6   (*Continued*)

Author (date)	Data and source (method)	Estimated elasticities	
		Price	Income
Porter (1986)	U.S. time series 1947–1982 per capita consumption Data sources are the same as Schneider, Klein, and Murphy (1981) (two-stage least squares)	−0.051 to −0.290	−0.095 to −0.167
Baltagi and Goel (1987)	U.S. state tax increases 1956–1983 The Tobacco Institute Lyon and Simon's (1968) method (quasi-experimental method)	−0.114 to −0.917	
Kao and Tremblay (1988)	U.S. time series 1953–1980 U.S. Department of Agriculture U.S. Bureau of the Census Bishop and Yoo (1985) (two-stage least squares)	−0.495 to −1.019	0.737 to 1.482
Russo (1989)	U.S. micro cross section 1980 National Health Interview Survey U.S. National Center for Health Statistics Tobacco Tax Council (tobit maximum likelihood)	−0.573	0.067
Chaloupka (1991)	National Health and Nutrition Examination Survey, 1976–1980 (two-stage least squares)	−0.37 to −0.27 (long-run)	
Wasserman et al. (1991)	National Health Interview Study, 1970–1985 Tobacco Institute price data (generalized linear model)	−0.283 to 0.059 (1988) (1976)	−0.038 to 0.051 (1988) (1976)
Keller, Hu, and Barnett (1991)	California Monthly Time Series Data, Jan. 1980–Jan. 1990 (instrumental variables)	−0.35 (pretax) −0.65 (posttax)	

Source: Russo (1989), Table 14, with both additions and updates by the author.

The elasticity estimates that have greater pertinence for our analysis of the role of excise taxes are the price elasticity estimates reported in Table 5–6. These estimates are based on studies utilizing a wide variety of data sources. Some of these analyses utilize cross-sectional data at a single point in time and base the elasticity estimates on differences in demand pattern observed in different locales that have different cigarette prices. Another group of studies is time series in nature, in which the changes in cigarette prices over time influence the shifting demand for cigarette products. The studies span a broad range of time periods, beginning in 1913 and including periods as recent as 1985. The data examined also pertain to both the United States and the United Kingdom.

Despite the diversity of approaches in the studies summarized in Table 5–6, most of the demand elasticities are clustered in the range from [−0.4 to −1.0].

Perhaps most strikingly, every study in the table was able to generate estimates that indicated a negative elasticity of demand for cigarettes. As one would expect with a normal economic good, the demand curve for cigarettes slopes downward; as the price of cigarettes declines, consumers increase their demand for the product. Similarly, price increases for cigarettes will reduce consumer demand.

These effects are particularly great in the case of teenagers, who appear to be most sensitive to the price. The evidence is, however, somewhat mixed, as some studies indicate greater price responsiveness by teenagers (e.g., Lewit, Coate, and Grossman [1981]) and other studies indicate no difference between teenagers and adults (e.g., Wasserman et al. [1991]). No studies suggest that teenagers are less responsive to prices than adults. These studies have not yet distinguished whether the greater responsiveness of teenagers stems from their differing financial status or the fact that this group constitutes new smokers as opposed to longer-term smokers.

The price responsiveness of cigarette demand implies that smoking decisions satisfy a basic but fairly undemanding test of rationality. It also highlights the potential role of taxes as a policy instrument for influencing cigarette smoking behavior. In particular, higher taxes will reduce the demand for cigarettes in much the same way as would higher risk perceptions. One can profitably analyze the potential role of taxes by making this linkage and assessing how excise taxes could be used to promote correct risk-taking decisions.

In situations of market failure involving goods traded on the market, a frequently suggested remedy for market failure is the use of taxes. Thus, economists have long suggested injury taxes for on-the-job injuries and various kinds of pollution taxes and marketable pollution-rights schemes for pollution. In the same vein, Harris (1980) has suggested the imposition of taxes on tar and nicotine content of cigarettes as a mechanism for internalizing these risks. The underlying supposition in his analysis is that smokers fail to perceive any health costs of smoking, which is clearly not the case empirically but which nevertheless provides a useful reference point for thinking about the economic consequences of a cigarette tax. Unlike an informational transfer effort, however, taxes will discourage the consumption of all consumers, not simply those who underassess the risk. These tax approaches have a direct analogue in the case of cigarettes, as one could impose a tax on cigarettes to discourage consumption in much the same manner as would be accomplished through higher risk perceptions.

Such a tax could address both the private and social costs of smoking. A recent analysis by Manning et al. (1989) explicitly addresses whether taxes on cigarettes and alcohol are sufficient to cover the external costs generated. Their analysis did not include the effects of secondhand smoke, but it did recognize important cost categories such as the pension and insurance costs of smoking. Smoking increases the rate of premature death for smokers. These adverse health effects impose health costs, many of which are shared through private and public health insurance programs. From a societal standpoint, premature death also lowers other insurance costs, notably the costs of pension benefits and social security. Determining whether the medical cost losses are greater than the annuity cost savings is not a simple matter because the timing of the losses differ: Medical cost savings occur at an earlier date.

The net loss on savings is governed by the relative weight one places on effects at different points in time—in particular, on the interest rate one uses to discount future losses. Low rates of discount place substantial weight on the annuity savings, so that there may be no net cost to society, excluding the costs of secondhand smoke. At real (i.e., inflation-adjusted) interest rates below 3.5 percent the net effect of smoking is to save society costs since the reduced pension and social security costs from premature death exceed the value of the increased medical expenses. At real rates of discount in excess of this amount, the burden on society becomes positive because of the reduced weight that will be placed on the deferred pension and social security savings.[12]

In the late 1980s and early 1990s the real rates of return to interest became distorted because the Federal Reserve Board had to exercise substantial monetary restraint in the presence of the high budgetary deficits. Thus, the U.S. economy experienced aberrationally high real rates of return on U.S. Treasury bills in the range of 3 percent. Nevertheless, these rates are sufficiently high to indicate that on balance smoking saves society insurance costs. Furthermore, econometric studies indicate that the long-run increase in productivity of the United States is below that level, which is consistent with an assumption that the net costs imposed by cigarettes on society are in fact negative.[13] Because the external costs and benefits of smoking to the rest of society are approximately offsetting, this component of the impacts of smoking will be ignored. Instead, I will focus on the private costs associated with the risk to the smoker rather than on the social costs.

Table 5–7 summarizes the excise tax percentage of cigarette prices by state, where these rates range from 20.3 percent in Virginia to 41.1 percent in Oregon. The national average is 30.8 percent, so that by any standard cigarettes are a heavily taxed commodity.

The objective of this analysis is to establish the risk equivalent of these excise taxes. In particular, what is the equivalent lung cancer risk perception endowment that establishes the same effect on smoking probabilities as does the cigarette excise tax?[14] This measure will provide a useful index of the degree to which taxes discourage consumption.

To establish this equivalence one needs an estimate of the price elasticity of cigarette purchases. Four such elasticities are used in the calculations in Table 5–7, where these elasticities range from −0.4 to −1.4. This range spans most of the elasticity estimates in the literature summarized in Table 5.6, with most estimates falling in the −0.4 to −1.0 range and higher elasticities such as −1.4 being reported for teenagers.[15]

The results of the excise tax simulation in Table 5–7 are quite striking. Even for the lowest elasticity column the risk equivalent of the excise tax greatly exceeds estimates of the "true" lung cancer risk, with the risk equivalent being 0.17 nationally. The effects increase almost proportionally in the other elasticity cases.

The principal economic implication of these results is quite strong. Even if

Table 5–7 Risk equivalent of 1985 smoking excise taxes by state

State	Taxes as a percent of retail price	Risk equivalent of cigarette excise taxes			
		$\epsilon = -0.4$	$\epsilon = -0.7$	$\epsilon = -1.0$	$\epsilon = -1.4$
Alabama	31.6	.17	.28	.38	.52
Alaska	29.1	.16	.26	.36	.48
Arizona	29.1	.16	.26	.36	.48
Arkansas	35.7	.19	.31	.43	.58
California	24.9	.14	.23	.31	.42
Colorado	32.6	.18	.29	.40	.53
Connecticut	35.4	.19	.31	.43	.57
Delaware	28.5	.16	.26	.35	.47
District of Columbia	26.5	.15	.24	.33	.44
Florida	32.5	.18	.29	.39	.53
Georgia	28.0	.16	.25	.35	.47
Hawaii	36.7	.20	.32	.44	.59
Idaho	25.1	.14	.23	.31	.42
Illinois	25.8	.15	.24	.32	.43
Indiana	28.3	.16	.26	.35	.47
Iowa	40.1	.21	.35	.48	.64
Kansas	38.8	.21	.34	.46	.62
Kentucky	22.2	.13	.21	.28	.38
Louisiana	30.4	.17	.27	.37	.50
Maine	39.0	.21	.34	.46	.63
Maryland	31.1	.17	.28	.38	.51
Massachusetts	36.5	.20	.32	.44	.59
Michigan	34.9	.19	.31	.42	.57
Minnesota	33.5	.18	.30	.41	.55
Mississippi	32.1	.18	.28	.39	.53
Missouri	28.5	.16	.26	.35	.47
Montana	31.4	.17	.28	.38	.52
Nebraska	32.7	.18	.29	.40	.53
Nevada	29.1	.16	.26	.36	.48
New Hampshire	33.0	.18	.29	.40	.54
New Jersey	35.8	.19	.31	.43	.58
New Mexico	27.7	.16	.25	.34	.46
New York	33.3	.18	.29	.40	.54
North Carolina	21.5	.13	.20	.27	.37
North Dakota	32.6	.18	.29	.40	.53
Ohio	30.6	.17	.27	.37	50
Oklahoma	32.5	.18	.29	.39	.53
Oregon	41.1	.21	.35	.49	.66
Pennsylvania	32.4	.18	.29	.39	.53
Rhode Island	38.7	.21	.34	.46	.62
South Carolina	25.9	.15	.24	.32	.43
South Dakota	35.9	.19	.31	.43	.58

(*continued*)

Table 5–7 (*Continued*)

State	Taxes as a percent of retail price	Risk equivalent of cigarette excise taxes			
		$\epsilon = -0.4$	$\epsilon = -0.7$	$\epsilon = -1.0$	$\epsilon = -1.4$
Tennessee	29.4	.16	.26	.36	.49
Texas	34.6	.19	.30	.42	.56
Utah	27.1	.15	.25	.34	.45
Vermont	31.5	.17	.28	.38	.52
Virginia	20.3	.12	.19	.26	.35
Washington	31.0	.17	.28	.38	.51
West Virginia	31.7	.17	.28	.39	.52
Wisconsin	37.0	.20	.32	.44	.60
Wyoming	24.5	.14	.23	.31	.41
National average	30.8	.17	.27	.38	.51

individuals had no awareness of lung cancer risks at all and assessed the risks as being zero, excise taxes would have discouraged smoking by more than the effect of accurate risk perceptions. The effect of taxes is to augment the role of lung cancer risk perceptions by roughly half to more than double, depending on the price elasticity of demand. Whether these taxes are sufficient to offset other risk perception inadequacies is less clear-cut since the level of the other risks from smoking are not as well established.

Based on the estimates in Lewit, Coate, and Grossman (1981), teenagers have the greatest price sensitivity at the high end of the range in Table 5–6, so that taxes serve as a particular discouragement to their smoking behavior. Excise taxes create the same decrease in smoking as would viewing the lung cancer risk as roughly a fifty-fifty proposition. This strong effect of excise taxes augments the already substantial role of the AGE16–21 group's above-average risk perceptions, which average .49. The combined effect of excise taxes and the lung cancer risk perceptions on smoking behavior is comparable to what would be observed if the younger members of the sample viewed lung cancer as roughly a certain outcome of smoking.

The strength of this effect hinges on the price responsiveness of teenagers. If teenagers exhibit only the same responsiveness as do adults, as is found in the more recent study by Wasserman et al. (1991), then the effects of taxes in discouraging consumption will be comparable to that for adults.[16]

TASTES, ADDICTION, AND ETHICS

There are a variety of reasons why some people choose to smoke whereas others do not. First, some people may have a stronger preference for the pleasures derived from smoking than do others. Differences in tastes influence the purchase of almost all economic commodities, whether they be cigarettes, automobiles, or books. Systematic differences in preferences will contribute to many of the observed patterns of smoking. A second contributor to the difference in the propensity to smoke is the character of individual risk perceptions. Individuals with a lower assessment of the smoking risk will be more attracted to smoking because the expected cost will be perceived as being lower. In the case of lung cancer we found that there were some differences of this type, although the discrepancy is not stark. Overall, smokers assess the lung cancer risk as being .37, which is .06 lower than the societal perception of .43.

The third contributor to differences in smoking rates is a difference in the tradeoffs people are willing to make between risks and other valued attributes of their choices. What drives smoking decisions is not simply the preference for smoking and the perception of the smoking risk, but also the rate at which individuals are willing to trade off higher risks for the smoking pleasures. More specifically, there may be a difference in the tradeoff between risks and other valued attributes of the commodity.

Table 5–8 provides a series of profiles of cigarette smokers and other health-related consumption activities. Smoking behavior and health practices generally are not random events. The age-related variations in smoking behavior are not substantial for the age-groups from 18 to 64, as smoking rates peak at 34.5 percent for the middle-age cohort. In contrast, heavy drinking is most prevalent among younger age-groups, and the propensity to be overweight increases with age. Men are more likely to smoke and to be heavy drinkers.

The effects of greatest interest are the role of income and education, which are a good measure of lifetime wealth. Smoking rates decline as education level increases. With a strong positive income elasticity of the demand for good health, one would expect the more affluent respondents to take greater health precautions of various kinds. Moreover, there may also be a class-based character to various activities. Smoking and drinking may have greater social acceptability in particular contexts. Knowledge of health risks also is positively correlated with education levels.[17]

These apparent differences in the tradeoffs that people make with respect to risk can be used to establish an index of individual willingness to bear risk. Because of the multiplicity of such metrics, the tradeoff that economists usually focus on is the risk-dollar tradeoff of the individual. This metric incorporates the individual's attitude toward expected health losses, while at the same time using the metric of money to establish a quantitative reference point for assessing the value of fostering of individual health relative to other aspects of one's consumption.

The main source of evidence that economists have used to analyze risk-dollar tradeoffs has been drawn from the labor market. Since the time of Adam Smith, economists have observed that workers will demand an extra premium to work on a job that poses additional risk. These compensating differentials are often quite large—on the order of several hundred dollars per year for the average blue-collar worker. Since this compensation is embedded within the entire structure of wages that is paid in the economy and is not always formalized in a collective bargaining agreement, one must use standard statistical techniques in

Table 5-8 Profile of personal health practices, 1985

Characteristic	Current smoker	Less physically active than contemporaries	Had 5 or more drinks on any one day[a]	30 Percent or more above desirable weight[b]
All persons[c]	30.1	16.4	37.5	13.0
AGE				
18–29 years old	31.9	17.1	54.4	7.5
30–44 years old	34.5	18.3	39.0	13.6
45–64 years old	31.6	15.3	24.6	18.1
65 years old and over	16.0	13.5	12.2	13.2
65–74 years old	19.7	15.8	NA	14.9
74 years old and over	10.0	9.8	NA	10.3
SEX				
Male	32.6	16.5	49.3	12.1
Female	27.8	16.3	23.3	13.7
RACE				
White	29.6	16.7	38.3	12.4
All other	33.1	14.3	29.9	16.4
Black	34.9	13.9	29.3	18.7
Other	24.8	16.5	33.3	6.7
EDUCATION LEVEL				
Less than 12 years	35.4	12.3	35.9	17.5
12 years	33.4	16.5	38.9	13.4
More than 12 years	23.1	19.1	36.8	9.4
FAMILY INCOME				
Less than $7,000	31.1	13.5	NA	16.1
$7,000 to $14,999	33.4	14.7	NA	15.3
$15,000 to $24,999	32.2	16.8	NA	13.4
$25,000 to $39,999	30.0	17.2	NA	12.1
$40,000 or more	25.2	19.4	NA	9.4

Source: U.S. Department of Commerce (1989).

[a] Percent of drinkers who had 5 or more drinks on any one day in the past year.

[b] Based on 1960 Metropolitan Life Insurance Company standards. Data are self-reported.

[c] Excludes persons whose health practices are unknown.

conjunction with information on employment patterns and worker risk levels to evaluate the levels of these premiums.

A useful index for putting these premiums in perspective is to analyze the compensation one receives per statistical injury. A considerable literature has evolved analyzing the value of a statistical life, which pertains to the compensation received per expected death in the workplace. In addition, workers also receive compensation for other aspects of the job.

The outcome that we will focus on here is the compensation workers receive for each average lost workday injury that they expect to experience on the job. This criticism applies to all injuries sufficiently severe to lead the worker to miss one or more days of work. The primary matter of interest is whether smokers differ from nonsmokers in terms of the implicit values they attach to expected injuries. For each expected injury that a worker faces in his or her job, how does the compensation one requires to bear this injury vary with smoking status? This concept is consequently an *ex ante* approach to the valuation of prospective statistical injuries rather than the *ex post* value of injuries already experienced. If smokers are willing to engage in their smoking behavior because they do in fact have a lower rate of tradeoff between the expected health costs of smoking and the other valued attributes of smoking consumption, then one would expect there to be a lower observed wage premium required by smokers to face job risks. Such evidence would constitute a consistency and rationality check on the earlier results since it would indicate that smokers differ systematically from nonsmokers in terms of their valuation of the health effects of smoking. Thus, their smoking status could be viewed as part of the rational self-selection into smoking behavior that is generated by a difference in tastes with respect to attitudes toward the valuation of risk.

Table 5–9 summarizes the estimates by Hersch and Viscusi (1990) of the implicit values per expected lost workday injury for a sample of 193 workers in the state of Oregon. We developed a new sample for this study so as to have a meaningful measure of the workers' job risk on a continuous risk scale that was pertinent to the workers' individual position. Moreover, the survey was designed to elicit information on cigarette smoking status as well as seat belt use, which is another form of behavior influencing one's individual risk. Use of seat belts and

Table 5–9   Implicit value of a lost workday injury

Equation	Group	Implicit value of a lost workday injury ($ per statistical injury)
1	Full sample	47,900
2	Smokers	26,100
2	Seat belt users	78,200
2	Nonsmoker–non-seat belt user	37,800
2	Smoker–seat belt user	66,400
3	Smoker–non-seat belt user	26,900
3	Nonsmoker–seat belt user	83,200
3	Nonsmoker–non-seat belt user	37,800
3	Smoker–seat belt user	71,200

Source: Based on Hersch and Viscusi (1990), Table 7. The risk variables included are the following (denote the job risk variable by Injury). Equation 1 included Injury; equation 2 included Injury, Injury × Cigarettes, Injury × Seat Belt Use; and equation 3 included Injury, Injury × Cigarettes, Injury × Seat Belt Use, and Injury × Cigarettes × Seat Belt Use. Cigarettes is equal to the number of cigarettes smoked by the respondent in an average day.

smoking both should reflect the same kinds of influence of individuals' attitudes toward expected health effects.

Table 5–9 reports the results for three different equations that have been estimated. In each case the dependent variable was the natural logarithm of the worker's wage, and the equation included a variety of measures of the worker's demographic characteristics and job attributes. Among the explanatory variables were the worker's age, race, sex, years of experience on the job, a series of six variables capturing the nonpecuniary characteristics of the job (e.g., repetitive work task), and union status. Based on the first equation, which includes a job risk variable that is not interacted with any other activities, the most one can infer is the average premium workers receive per lost workday injury. The second equation includes interaction terms of the job risk with the amount of cigarette smoking (number of cigarettes smoked per day) and seat belt use (yes or no), thus making it possible to ascertain the implicit values of injuries received by smokers, seat belt users, and people who neither smoke nor wear seat belts. The third equation estimated makes it possible to analyze the richest set of variations since it adds to the variables in equation 2 an interactive effect of job risks with cigarette smoking, seat belt use, and both smoking and seat belt use. As a consequence, one can break out a more detailed set of population groups that are of interest.

Table 5–9 summarizes the dollar wage compensation received per statistical job injury. For the full sample, workers overall require compensation for injuries that reflects wage compensation of $47,900 for each expected workday injury. Since the workers in the sample assess their annual probability of a lost workday injury as being 1/17 on average, the compensation received by each worker per year for this additional risk was approximately $2,800, controlling for other aspects of the worker and his or her job.

The variation of this implicit value of job injuries with respect to smoking status follows the expected pattern. Equation 2 in Table 5–9 indicates that smokers value injuries at just over half the value attached by the full sample, as they are willing to bear an expected workplace injury for $26,100.

In contrast, one should expect that seat belt users would demand higher prices per unit risk because their act of wearing a seat belt has revealed the high value they attach to the potential health losses of a motor vehicle accident. This relationship is in fact borne out, as the results for equation 2 indicate that seat belt users receive compensation for the job risks they bear on the order of $78,200 for each job accident.

The findings for the various combinations of smokers and seat belt use in equation 3 of Table 5–9 are similar in nature. In each case, smoking status lowers the valuation and seat belt use raises the valuation from its counterpart. Of all the population groups considered, smokers overall and smokers who do not wear seat belts attach the lowest implicit value to injuries—about $26,000. The differences between these two groups are not statistically significant. This result is consistent with differences in individual tastes driving choices in a rational economic manner.

When considering any empirical result such as this, it is useful to explore other possible explanations. Since these estimates are based on actual earnings premiums that workers received for the risks they face, there is no potential problem of workers misrepresenting the wage compensation they must receive. The one subjective component of the survey that depended on individual worker responses was the risk assessment for the job on which they work. However, could seemingly consistent results on attitudes toward risk arise if the same people who underestimated smoking risks also underestimated job risks, leading them to engage in both sets of risky activities without good information? To the extent that any effect such as this is at work, it will tend to lead to a *higher* estimated implicit value of an injury for smokers and nonseat belt users than was observed in the table. In particular, an underestimate of the job risk for these groups will lead to a higher estimated value of their wage compensation per unit risk that they assess, thus increasing the estimated implicit value of an injury. Systematic neglect of the risk through underestimation of it consequently cannot account for the disparity in the observed rates of tradeoff.

These results are also consistent with estimates of the implicit value of life revealed through smoking decisions. Ippolito and Ippolito (1984) estimate that for their 1980 sample of individuals, the average value of life-saving by the shift in smoking behavior as a result of the dissemination of cigarette-health disclosures was in the range of $300,000 to $600,000. Since the life years at stake are deferred and involve fewer expected years of life lost than would result from the typical fatal job accident, value-of-life estimates of this magnitude are quite reasonable and are at the low end of the value-of-life estimates in the literature.[18] Their estimates are consequently consistent with the implicit value of injury estimates derived above.

What we find is that the revealed preferences of smokers with respect to the value of expected health impacts are quite consistent with those revealed in their smoking behavior. As a consequence, although there was a minor disparity in the perceptions of smokers and nonsmokers, it is largely other factors such as differences in tastes that drive the differences in smoking decisions.

One might, of course, question at a very fundamental level whether the tastes revealed in individual decisions are sound or whether we should try to influence these tastes. One might view the activities of the Surgeon General as not only providing information to people but also trying to increase the value they attach to their health. Changing fundamental preferences is typically quite difficult.[19] Moreover, most economic analyses usually treat tastes as given aspects of individual behavior, not parameters that can be manipulated. In many cases we may appear to be influencing tastes, whereas in fact we are simply providing information about the welfare implications of products that enable people to think more sensibly about the benefits they will derive from consumption of them.

Even if we could influence tastes through government policy or some other action, it is not clear that we should do so. Imposing the preferences of policymakers on the citizenry at large is inconsistent with the democratic principles that underlie economic analyses of the proper role of the government. The task of the government is to maximize the net benefits to the citizenry as they perceive these effects, not as they would perceive them if their preferences were more similar to those of government officials.

One main exception to respecting individual choices occurs in situations in which these choices are not well informed. In that context, maximizing the expected welfare of the citizenry based on the actual probabilities of different outcomes rather than on the misperceived chances is a more sensible approach to policy.

CONCLUSION

From an economic standpoint, cigarette smoking can be viewed as a potentially hazardous consumption activity. When viewed in this manner, the fundamental question is whether decisions are made rationally. Perception of the risks influences smoking behavior, as one would expect based on an economic model of risky consumption behavior. Moreover, these smoking decisions are consistent with other individual risk-taking activities, such as willingness to bear job risks in return for wage compensation. The role of excise taxes serves to discourage consumption in much the same manner as would increasing lung cancer risk perceptions by as much as 50 to 100 percent, depending on the price sensitivity of the demand for cigarettes. Cigarette excise taxes do more to reduce smoking propensities than would elimination of any proclivities toward smoking stemming from underestimation of the potential lung cancer hazards. The influence of lung cancer risk perceptions on smoking behavior provides striking evidence of the importance of individual responses to risk.

NOTES

1. See Peltzman (1975) and Blomquist (1988).

2. See, among others, Thaler and Rosen (1979) and Viscusi (1979).

3. The only study of wage responses to subjective job risk perceptions using a continuous risk measure is that of Viscusi and O'Connor (1984). The first study using a 0–1 measure of subjective risk perceptions is Viscusi (1979).

4. *New York Times*, May 17, 1988, p. A1. For more detail see also U.S. Department of Health and Human Services (1988). Earlier Surgeon General's reports dealing with cigarettes containing higher levels of nicotine than those now marketed specifically disavowed the addiction notion: "The tobacco habit should be characterized as an habituation rather than an addiction." U.S. Department of Health, Education and Welfare (1964), p. 34. For evidence on the decreased nicotine content of cigarettes, see U.S. Department of Health and Human Services (1983), p. 372.

5. See Stigler and Becker (1977), Schelling (1984), and Becker and Murphy (1988) for discussions of the addiction phenomenon from different perspectives.

6. This point is discussed in Viscusi (1979) with respect to transactions costs of changing jobs that are risky and have uncertain properties.

7. For an articulation of such views, see Goodin (1989) and Warner (1986).

8. To model the discrete cigarette smoking decision, consider the following simple one-period model. Let there be two states of the world, life and death. When alive, the individual reaps a utility U(Smoke) if he smokes and U(Don't) if he doesn't smoke. Death offers a payoff V, and the probability of death is s if one smokes and 0 otherwise. An individual will choose to smoke if

$$(1 - s)U(Smoke) + sV > U(Don't),$$

or

$$[U(Smoke) - U(Don't)] + s[V - U(Don't)] > 0.$$

The first term in the first of these equations represents the net utility gain from cigarette smoking, which reflects both taste factors and prices, and the second term represents the expected utility loss from death. Let us parameterize the second equation with a linear model, letting β_i (i=1,2) be the coefficent vectors, Y_1 be a vector of taste and price variables, Y_2 be a vector of variables affecting utility loss, and u_2 be a random error term. The smoking decision is attractive if

$$\beta_1 Y_1 + \beta_2 s Y_2 + u_2 > 0,$$

or

$$pr(Smoke) = [pr(\beta_1 Y_1 + \beta_2 s Y_2 > - u_2] = [1 + exp(-\beta_1 Y_1 - \beta_2 s Y_2)]^{-1}$$

if we assume a logistic probability distribution.

9. Following the same procedure as in Chapter 4, the test coefficients (standard errors) are −0.1601 (0.2471) for equation 1, −0.1564 (0.2469) for equation 2, 0.0040 (0.1754) for equation 3, and 0.0071 (0.1753) for equation 4, easily passing the endogeneity test in all four cases. The test of overidentifying restrictions for the excluded instruments is also passed.

10. The standard approach typified by the early study by Thaler and Rosen (1976) and reflected in almost all subsequent analyses is to focus on the death risk of jobs. Viscusi (1979) extended these measures to also include nonfatal risks and subjective risk perceptions, but not all sources of risk have been recognized by such studies.

11. In the standard errors in variables problem, the true risk s_i for person i is given by

$$s_i = RISK_i + u_i.$$

One can obtain efficient estimates that reduce the resulting bias through a two-stage least squares procedure in which RISK is replaced by an instrumental variable estimator. In particular, the instruments used to construct the estimated value of RISK were a series of fifty regional dummy variables, following the approach in Friedman (1957), and a 0–1 variable for whether RISK was above or below its median value, as suggested by Wald (1940). These results appear in Table 5–4.

12. These savings have also been documented by Shoven, Sundberg, and Bunker (1987). More generally, see Tollison and Wagner (1988) for a broader discussion of the social costs and benefits of smoking.

13. See Baumol (1986) and Darby (1984) for estimates that the annual increase in labor productivity in the United States has been in the 1.5 to 2.25 percent range.

14. More specifically, the RISK increment $\Delta RISK_i$ for individual i has the same effect as current excise taxes, or

$$pr(Smoke_i | Risk_i, Excise\ Tax_i) =$$
$$pr(Smoke_i | Risk_i + \Delta Risk_i, Excise\ Tax_i = 0),$$

where this equality is maintained using the results from estimates of the equations in Table 5–3.

15. See the studies by Lewit and Coate (1982), Russo (1987), Comanor and Wilson (1974), and Schmalensee (1972).

16. These differences across studies depend in part on the inclusion of a smoking regulation variable in Wasserman et al. (1991).

17. See Kenkel (1991).

18. See Viscusi (1983).

19. The failure of such efforts is documented by Adler and Pittle (1984).

6

Individual Learning and Age Variations in Risk Perceptions and Smoking Decisions

From the standpoint of market failure with respect to individual decisions under uncertainty, smoking behavior raises two classes of issues. First, do individuals understand the potential risks posed by their smoking decisions? Second, if they do understand these risks, do they take them into account when deciding whether they will smoke?

These concerns are particularly acute in the case of younger individuals, since most smokers initiate their smoking behavior when they are relatively young. In view of the considerable attention that has been focused on the costs associated with cessation of smoking, which the Surgeon General has designated as a problem of addiction,[1] it becomes particularly important to determine whether young cigarette smokers understand the risks and act upon these risk perceptions in a responsible manner.

The issue of cigarette addiction has become prominent in the economic literature as well. Two principal schools of thought have developed. Schelling (1984) hypothesizes that the addiction issue represents an internal battle for self-control. There are competing selves within the individual, and the question is whether the individual will succeed in taking the actions that promote his or her long-term interests as opposed to those that simply promote one's more immediate preferences. In Schelling's view, the task of the smoker is one of a battle to impose intertemporal rationality on one's decisions. Another school of thought has developed pertaining to models of rational addiction in which individuals voluntarily choose an addictive consumption path. These models have been espoused by Becker and Murphy (1988).[2]

Although neither of these treatments focuses in detail on the risk attributes of the product, risk concerns are clearly central to how one interprets each of the models. In the case of irrational addiction, the concern with addictive behavior will be less if individuals are fully cognizant of the results of their addictive behavior at the time they begin their addiction and if they fully understand the character of their future preferences. Does the 20-year-old smoker fully recognize how his or her future self will value health as compared with smoking? A 20-year-old may begin an addictive habit with the intention of quitting at age 40, knowing it will be difficult to do so. If smokers know in advance what all the consequences of their actions will be, including the character of their future preferences, then economists would argue that the resulting outcomes are efficient. One way in which the battle for self-control could lead to an inefficient outcome is if consumers initially underestimate the risks posed by smoking, subsequently wish to alter this consumption pattern, and then realize they have made a mistake that cannot be easily corrected. The welfare loss from these mistakes will not exceed the costs of change, however, so that they are not unbounded.

In the case of rational models of addiction, one cannot argue that these addiction decisions are in fact truly rational unless there is some understanding of the risks involved. Analysis of the underlying risk perceptions is consequently central to ascertaining the welfare consequences of behavior that has come under the general heading of addiction, even though our focus on cross-sectional data with single period choices is not ideally suited to analyzing the process of changes in smoking behavior patterns.

The fact that many smokers profess a desire to quit smoking should not necessarily be treated as an index of market failure. Almost half of the residents of Los Angeles indicate a desire to move out of the city, but do not do so.[3] Almost one-third of all blue-collar workers would like to leave their jobs but do not.[4] Statements such as these may indicate that there is some dissatisfaction with one or more attributes of a particular product or activity. Survey statements in which individuals indicate that they would like to quit smoking, for example, might mean that they would like to smoke without risk. However, the fact that they have continued to smoke even with the availability of chewing gum with nicotine suggests that these statements concerning a desire to quit should not always be taken at face value. Fortunately, there has been a wave of recent empirical work focusing on the extent to which these costs of change are of consequence.[5] The discussion below is intended to address an important aspect of these decisions, notably the level of risk perceptions and, in particular, the extent to which these risk perceptions vary with individual age. More specifically, are younger individuals incapable of making sound smoking decisions, which will ultimately affect their long-run smoking behavior?

Evidence from other risk contexts does not inspire complete confidence in these decision-making capabilities. Younger drivers lead all age-groups in motor vehicle fatality rates, where a major component of these accidents is attributable to teenage drunken driving.[6] Recall from Table 5–8 that individuals age 18–29 also are much more likely to have had five or more drinks on any one day in one year. Moreover, in terms of the total risk of death from accidents, individuals age 15–24 have a higher risk level than any other age-group except the elderly, who are susceptible to injuries from falls.[7] If a proclivity toward risk-taking behavior in this decision context is reflected in others as well, then we would expect to find evidence of inadequate risk perceptions and failure to respond to risks when examining the smoking decisions of younger individuals.

An offsetting influence is that the mix of the information received by younger age-groups will incorporate more adverse information with respect to the consequences of smoking. Public dissemination of risk information has been widespread, particularly over the past two decades. Moreover, the increased social controversy with respect to smoking has created heightened social awareness. One would expect that individuals whose experiences have been dominated by this more recent climate would have higher risk perceptions than those with a longer-term perspective.

Studies by psychologists utilizing the kinds of qualitative risk-perception questions analyzed in Chapter 3 indicate that even very young children have negative attitudes toward smoking. Table 6–1 reports the results by Schneider and Vanmastrig (1974) assessing the risk perceptions of children age 7–8, 10–11, and 13–14. The results are similar for each of these age-groups, and for concreteness we will focus on the youngest age-group represented in the sample. Over 99 percent of all children age 7–8 believe that smoking can cause cancer, and an almost equal number believe that smoking shortens a person's life.[8] The overwhelming majority of children also believe that it is very hard to stop smoking. Whether children wouldn't smoke if adults stopped smoking depends largely on the age of the child. A striking result in Table 6–1 is that by the early teen years there is a dramatic drop in the influence of parental example on the child's attitude toward smoking. This pattern may reflect the greater independence of this age-group. The level of awareness of smoking risks is quite substantial, and one would expect this awareness to be translated into risk perceptions in much the same way that the public opinion poll results were also mirrored in the quantitative risk assessments discussed in Chapter 4.

This chapter will utilize the national survey of smoking risk perceptions and smoking behavior to investigate the role of individual age with respect to smoking behavior. These data will enable us to analyze smoking behavior as a case study in the economics of potentially risky consumption decisions. In particular, we will examine the level of subjective risk perceptions using probability assessments that make it possible to compare subjective perceptions with actual risk levels to determine the extent and direction of any bias. In addition, the results will illuminate the role of different sources of information by analyzing the variations in risk perception with age and smoking status. Finally, it will be

Table 6–1 Smoking experiences, beliefs, attitudes, and perception of attitudes of significant others by age-group

	Age		
Questions and statements	7–8 Years	10–11 Years	13–14 Years
Statements of belief (percentages of children responding "true")			
Smoking can cause cancer	99.2	100.0	99.0
Smoking shortens a person's life	96.7	99.2	88.1
It is very hard to stop smoking	74.8	74.2	76.2
Children wouldn't smoke if parents stopped smoking	79.2	75.2	43.4

Source: Schneider and Vanmastrig (1974), p. 74.

possible to assess how these risk perceptions are transmitted into smoking decisions, and to obtain a more refined assessment of the risk-taking process than in other choice contexts.[9]

After discussing the sample in the section on "Sample Characteristics," the "Patterns of Risk Perception" section uses detailed data on lung cancer risk perceptions to yield results that accord quite closely with the expected patterns of information acquisition. Overall, young respondents overestimate the level of lung cancer risks. "The Lung Cancer Risk-Perception Equation" section's analysis of the determinants of risk perception addresses the independent effect of variables, such as individual age. The linkage of smoking risks to smoking behavior for the age range 16–21 is not significantly different from that of older age-groups. Appendices 6A, 6B, and 6C articulate the learning model being tested more formally and present more detailed econometric results.

SAMPLE CHARACTERISTICS

The data base used for this analysis is the national survey of smoking behavior by Audits & Surveys used in Chapters 4 and 5. The primary age-group of interest here is the young age-group in the age range 16–21—11.3 percent of the sample. This age distribution captures the central age span during which smoking rates greatly increase—the latter teenage years.[10]

The central variable in the empirical analysis is the risk perception variable (RISK). The survey asked respondents how many of each group of 100 smokers would get lung cancer. Overall, 381 of the 3,119 individual respondents to the survey had missing RISK responses, or 11 percent of the sample. The nonrespondents were similar to those with valid RISK responses except that older individuals were less likely to answer the RISK question. The possibility of sample selection bias will be explicitly addressed in the results below.

PATTERNS OF RISK PERCEPTION

The pattern of risk perceptions in Table 6–2 follows the predictions of a rational learning model considered in Appendix 6A. The principal hypothesis is that younger age-groups should have the highest risk perceptions because the mix of their risk information is from a time period with increased smoking risk information. For each of the three smoking categories, the adult population group has lung cancer risk perceptions that are significantly lower than for the young age-group.[11] In addition, when one moves to the oldest sample group (AGE46+), the risk perception drops even more for current smokers, but for all respondent groups there is no significant decline in risk perceptions between the middle and oldest age-groups.[12] This diminishing effect of risk information is also consistent with a rational learning model.

The general pattern as one moves across the rows (from current smokers to former smokers and then to nonsmokers in any age-group) is that the risk percep-

Table 6–2 Variations in risk perceptions with age and smoking status

| Age-group | Mean RISK (standard error or mean) by group | | | |
	Current smoker	Former smoker	Nonsmoker	All respondents in age-group
AGE 16–21	.445	.429	.511	.490
	(.043)	(.037)	(.017)	(.015)
AGE 22–45	.382	.390	.454	.417
	(.011)	(.013)	(.010)	(.006)
AGE 46+	.328	.421	.456	.418
	(.017)	(.015)	(.011)	(.008)
All ages	.368	.408	.464	.426
	(.009)	(.010)	(.007)	(.005)

tion rises, which one would expect since we are moving toward groups with a higher proportion of their information coming in a stronger antismoking environment and in an era with more government provision of risk information.[13] The assessed risks in the scientific literature have risen over time as well. The only case where a rise does not occur (i.e., young current smokers have a higher risk assessment than young former smokers) involves a difference that is not statistically significant. Moreover, it is unclear which of the two groups has actually had more experience smoking cigarettes. The interpretation of the smoking status results is not as clear-cut as the age variations because smoking status is the result of a discretionary decision. Other explanations, such as cognitive dissonance and the self-selection of people with low risk assessments into smoking, are also possible.

Table 6–3 provides a more detailed perspective on the distribution of risk-perception levels. As is indicated by a comparison of the risk perceptions for the entire sample in all age-groups and for the younger individuals, the younger respondents tend to have higher risk perceptions than their more senior counterparts. In particular, younger individuals are more concentrated in the higher risk perception categories than older individuals. Moreover, for all smoking status groups, the AGE16–21 group has a significantly higher level of lung cancer risk perceptions.[14]

An interesting policy question is the extent to which individuals overestimate the risk. Thus, from the standpoint of market failure we are not concerned simply with the level of risk perceptions but with whether these perceptions are above or below the actual risk level. It should be emphasized that these assessments pertain only to the lung cancer risk, not to all risks of smoking. The overall smoking risk perception is what is pertinent for such broader policy judgments.[15]

Although the scientific basis for determining the lung cancer risk is not precise because of the difficult problems in tracking causality for diseases, our estimate in Chapter 4 using information provided by the Surgeon General indicated that the "true" lung cancer risk is in the range .05 to .10. Since Table 6–3 provides

Table 6–3 Distribution of risk perception for cigarette smoking, ages 16–21

Distribution of risk perceptions (RISK)	All age-groups	All respondents age 16–21	All smokers	Smokers age 16–21
RISK < .05	.052	.031	.092	.083
.05 ≤ RISK < .10	.046	.034	.051	.067
.10 ≤ RISK < .20	.117	.088	.130	.117
.20 ≤ RISK < .30	.136	.117	.146	.133
.30 ≤ RISK < .40	.090	.094	.114	.117
.40 ≤ RISK < .50	.052	.063	.050	.067
.50 ≤ RISK < .60	.239	.188	.228	.083
.60 ≤ RISK < .70	.070	.097	.056	.017
.70 ≤ RISK < .80	.084	.105	.050	.083
.80 ≤ RISK < .90	.042	.088	.027	.067
.90 ≤ RISK < 1.00	.041	.057	.028	.067
RISK = 1.00	.030	.037	.026	.100
Mean RISK	.426	.490	.368	.445
(standard error of mean)	(.005)	(.015)	(.009)	(.043)

detailed breakdowns by deciles, readers wishing to explore the sensitivity of the results to other reference risk levels can do so.

The overall implication of Table 6–3 is that individuals assess the lung cancer risks associated with smoking as being greater than the "true" risk level, and the extent of overestimation is particularly great for the youngest age cohort. Moreover, the asymmetry of risk perceptions around the "true" risk leads to overestimation that greatly exceeds risk underestimation. The net effect is that only a small segment of the sample underestimates the actual risk level. In the case of young cigarette smokers, under 10 percent of the sample believes that the risk is less than .05, and only 15 percent of the sample believes that the risk is less than .10, so that the overwhelming majority have risk assessments in excess of the estimated risk level.

The risk perceptions of those below the "true" risk level are quite different from those above. For respondents below the risk threshold of .05, the average value of RISK and its associated 95 percent confidence interval is .015 ± .001, whereas for respondents with RISK values greater than or equal to .05, the mean RISK and its associated 95 percent confidence interval is .449 ± .005. Similarly, with a risk threshold of .10, one obtains .034 ± .001 for risk underestimators and .468 ± .005 for those with RISK ≥ .10.

An intriguing aspect of Table 6–3 is the reasonably large fraction of smokers —10 percent of all young smokers—who believe the risk level is 1.0 yet continue to smoke. Although rational explanations involving the role of time lags and discounting are no doubt possible, another contributing factor is that the assessed cases of lung cancer per 100 smokers tend to be clustered at salient numbers. Respondents assessing a RISK of 1.0 may believe that lung cancer is highly likely but not necessarily a certain outcome.

THE LUNG CANCER RISK-PERCEPTION EQUATION

Table 6–4 reports several specifications of the lung cancer risk perception equation in which different sets of variables are included so as to distinguish the different influences at work. Appendix 6B details the statistical underpinnings of

Table 6–4 Lung cancer risk assessment equations[a]

Independent variables	Coefficients (standard errors)				
	1	2	3	4	5
Intercept	0.4362[b]	0.4790[b]	0.5175[b]	0.5250[b]	0.5143[b]
	(0.0172)	(0.0242)	(0.0246)	(0.0554)	(0.0354)
AGE 16–21	0.0736[b]	0.0711[b]	0.0546[b]	0.0554[b]	0.0497[b]
	(0.0170)	(0.0170)	(0.0170)	(0.0170)	(0.0217)
AGE 22–45	0.0028	−0.0004	−0.0004	0.0055	0.0011
	(0.0104)	(0.0105)	(0.0104)	(0.0104)	(0.0150)
MALE	−0.0564[b]	−0.0556[b]	−0.0489[b]	−0.0480[b]	−0.0484[b]
	(0.0100)	(0.0100)	(0.0099)	(0.0099)	(0.0100)
HOUSEHOLD SIZE	0.0041	0.0039	0.0032	0.0040	0.0037
	(0.0050)	(0.0051)	(0.0050)	(0.0050)	(0.0051)
PAST SMOKER OR SMOKER	—	—	−0.0681[b]	—	—
	—	—	(0.0097)	—	—
SMOKER (Instrumental Variable)	—	—	—	−0.0830[b]	−0.0827[b]
	—	—	—	(0.0164)	(0.0164)
PAST SMOKER (Instrumental Variable)	—	—	—	−0.0450[b]	−0.0447[b]
	—	—	—	(0.0107)	(0.0107)
LAMBDA (selectivity bias term)	—	—	—	—	0.0078
	—	—	—	—	(0.0187)
Ideas heard					
SHORTENS LIFE	—	−0.0079	−0.0084	−0.0123	−0.0123
		(0.0135)	(0.0134)	(0.0134)	(0.0134)
DANGEROUS TO HEALTH	—	−0.0237[b]	−0.0262[b]	−0.0272[b]	−0.0272[b]
		(0.0140)	(0.0138)	(0.0138)	(0.0138)
BAD, NOT DANGEROUS	—	−0.0382[b]	−0.0360[b]	−0.0362[b]	−0.0362[b]
		(0.0135)	(0.0134)	(0.0133)	(0.0133)
NOT BAD FOR HEALTH	—	0.0089	0.0051	0.0023	0.0021
		(0.0133)	(0.0132)	(0.0132)	(0.0132)
$\bar{R}^2$	.02	.02	.03	.05	.05

[a] Each equation also includes a series of 7 regional dummy variables.

[b] Denotes coefficients that are statistically significant at the 5 percent level, one-tailed test.

this analysis. The low explanatory power of all three equations in Table 6–4 suggests that factors other than those reflected in these demographic and broad informational variables largely account for smoking risk perceptions. The focus here is not on developing a predictive model but on testing specific hypotheses relating to respondent age.

Equation 1 in Table 6–4 includes only the background variables and regional dummy variables, which reflect differences in experience, the character of information that has been acquired, and regional price differences. The youngest age-group (AGE16–21) has higher risk perceptions, which is consistent with the earlier view that the smoking information the youngest cohort has received includes a much higher fraction of high-risk messages. The Surgeon General's efforts and the character of cigarette warnings have become more vigorous in recent years, and there has been a dramatic increase in social pressure against smoking. As predicted, the young will be more heavily affected by the recent antismoking campaigns. Males have a significantly lower risk perception on average. This pattern may reflect sex differences in attitudes toward risk or a difference in exposure to smoking. Men are more likely to be in contact with smokers than are women, so that they will have lower risk perceptions if these experiences provide indications of a lower risk than the antismoking campaign efforts. Both the YOUNG and MALE coefficients remain strongly significant in all five specifications, so that these effects are not attributable to the omission of other substantive variables.

Equation 2 of Table 6–4 adds a series of four variables that pertain to whether the individual has heard different statements about cigarette smoking, thus capturing the role of various forms of information that has been received. In particular, respondents were asked whether they had heard that "cigarette smoking will most likely shorten a person's life" (SHORTENS LIFE d.v.), "cigarette smoking is dangerous to a person's health" (DANGEROUS TO HEALTH d.v.), "cigarette smoking is bad for a person's health but not dangerous" (BAD, NOT DANGEROUS d.v.), and "cigarette smoking is not bad for a person's health" (NOT BAD FOR HEALTH d.v.).[16]

The four informational variables included in equation 2 of Table 6–4 have little effect on risk perceptions, which suggests that these statements have little informational content beyond what people already know. Two of the variables have coefficients that are not statistically significant, and the other two are of small magnitude. Somewhat surprisingly, the statement that is closest to the 1965 Surgeon General's warning (DANGEROUS TO HEALTH) is associated with a risk perception .02 lower than average. A somewhat greater negative discrepancy is observed for BAD, NOT DANGEROUS.

Equation 3 in Table 6–4 includes a dummy variable for whether the respondent has ever smoked either in the past or at present. Since this variable could potentially be endogenous, this possibility was tested formally and rejected.[17] The results for equation 3 in Table 6–4 indicate that past smoking has the expected negative effect on risk perceptions, as a history of smoking reduces the perceived RISK probability by .07.

Equations 4 and 5 in Table 6–4 report on estimates from the simultaneous equations system in which smoking status affects risk perceptions and one's risk assessment influences smoking status.[18] Both of the smoking status variables have significant negative effects on the risk assessment, as a CURRENT SMOKER will assess the lung cancer probability as being .08 lower and a PAST SMOKER will assess the probability as being .05 lower. Equation 5 adds the selectivity bias term LAMBDA, to control for potential bias that arises from some individuals not giving valid answers to the risk perception question. This variable, which is discussed more fully in Appendix 6B, is not statistically significant.

From a market failure standpoint one's main concern is not with the overall level of risk perception but with the probability that these perceptions are below the "true" risk. Thus, one could replace the dependent variable in equation 2 by the probability that the risk is underestimated. Such an assessment provides insight into the character of an important cigarette risk component but of course will not address all other smoking-related risks.

Table 6–5 presents logit estimates of the risk underestimation equation using

Table 6–5   Probability that individual underestimates the risk, logit model[a]

Independent variables	Coefficients (standard errors)			
	True risk = 0.05		True risk = 0.10	
	1	2	3	4
Intercept	−2.9914[b]	−4.0834[b]	−2.3041[b]	−3.0131[b]
	(0.3121)	(0.4548)	(0.2286)	(0.3332)
AGE 16–21	−0.7860[b]	−0.5142	−0.7429[b]	−0.5468[b]
	(0.3398)	(0.3462)	(0.2427)	(0.2470)
AGE 22–45	−0.3560	−0.3083	−0.4290[b]	−0.4003[b]
	(0.1720)	(0.1737)	(0.1294)	(0.1308)
MALE	0.5794[b]	0.4775[b]	0.5622[b]	0.4870[b]
	(0.1647)	(0.1660)	(0.1236)	(0.1246)
HOUSEHOLD SIZE	−0.0840	−0.0739	−0.0395	−0.0300
	(0.0937)	(0.0911)	(0.0669)	(0.0678)
PAST OR CURRENT SMOKER	—	0.8601[b]	—	0.6766[b]
		(0.1807)		(0.1302)
Ideas heard SHORTENS LIFE	—	−0.0671	—	0.0101
		(0.2214)		(0.1720)
DANGEROUS TO HEALTH	—	0.3614	—	0.2473
		(0.2290)		(0.1793)
BAD, NOT DANGEROUS	—	0.1263	—	−0.1208
		(0.2306)		(0.1677)
NOT BAD FOR HEALTH	—	0.1263	—	−0.1208
		(0.2246)		(0.1670)
Log likelihood	−615.16	−599.88	−968.83	−952.53

[a] Each equation also includes a set of 7 regional dummy variables.

[b] Denotes coefficients that are statistically significant at the 5 percent level, one-tailed test.

two different "true" lung cancer risk reference points—.05 and .10. The results are quite similar to the RISK perception equation. Sample members AGE 16–21 are less likely to underestimate the risk, and MALE sample members are more likely to underestimate the risk. Individuals with a smoking history are more likely to underestimate the risk, but the effect is fairly small.

It is particularly striking that none of the four informational variables has a statistically significant effect on risk underestimation. These results do not imply that knowledge is unimportant. Rather, they suggest that there is sufficiently widespread familiarity with the knowledge tested that this knowledge is uncorrelated with smoking risk perceptions.

AGE DIFFERENCES IN SMOKING BEHAVIOR

The costs associated with altering one's consumption behavior are of consequence only if there is a change in one's optimal consumption decision over time. One prominent source of change is individual learning. If individuals begin smoking at a young age because they underassess the risk and then subsequently increase their risk perceptions, there may be expected welfare benefits associated with quitting. The transactions costs associated with quitting may make this a costly process of learning and adaptation, so that there will be a welfare loss as compared with the situation of full information regarding the actual risk level. It is often suggested by critics of cigarettes that individuals become lured into smoking in this manner. The results in the sections "Risk Pattern Perception," and "The Lung-Cancer Risk Perception Equation," did not indicate any such age-related bias. In fact, the opposite bias was evident.

The risk-perception results do not in and of themselves eliminate the potential for irrational behavior by younger age-groups. Other potential health hazards of smoking and one's understanding of the costs of changing one's smoking behavior also influence any rationality judgment. Moreover, one must also show that this group acts upon these perceptions in making their smoking decisions.

Appendix 6C considers the role of age with respect to the influence of risk perceptions. The main result is that the risk perceptions of the young affect smoking perceptions to the same degree as for the older age-groups. Thus, there is no evidence of a dampening of the role of risk perceptions for younger age-groups. Since their level of risk perceptions for smoking is greater, the absence of any difference in the risk perceptions-smoking linkage implies that overall the presence of smoking risks discourages smoking more for younger age-groups than for their senior counterparts. There is certainly no evidence of greater neglect of smoking risks by the very young. Indeed, the opposite is the case, which is exactly what we would predict given their different informational environment.

CONCLUSION

The patterns of smoking and risk perceptions accord with one's expectations given the character of the risk information that has been provided. There has been a tremendous amount of recent publicity devoted to the hazards of smoking. Given the pronounced tendency to overestimate prominently publicized risks, this particular aspect of the smoking risk context should lead younger individuals to be particularly likely to overestimate smoking risks. This bias does not reflect a failure to process risk information accurately, as the typical form of government risk information transfer indicates that a hazard is present but does not indicate its specific probability.

The observed pattern of risk perceptions accords with what one would expect given the different mix of risk perceptions for different segments of the population. Most important is that the youngest age cohort has a high risk perception and is more likely to overestimate the risk than the population at large, which reflects this group's substantial reliance on recently provided information pertaining to the smoking risks.

The presence of substantial perceptions does not necessarily imply that the subsequent smoking decisions by younger individuals will be rational. Decisions could, for example, be unaffected by risk perceptions. The empirical evidence, however, indicates that perception of the risks influences smoking behavior, as one would expect based on an economic model of risky consumption behavior. Moreover, examination of the determinants of smoking behavior indicates that there is no statistically significant difference in the manner in which risk perceptions influence smoking behavior for the youngest age cohort. The net effect is that with higher risk perceptions and a similar behavioral response, there is no evidence of younger consumers being lured into smoking in any disproportionate manner.

These results contrast with the higher degrees of apparent irresponsibility of youths with respect to drunken driving. Moreover, they are also pertinent to welfare assessments of problems of smoking "addiction," since any welfare losses associated with costs of changing consumption behavior depend on the rationality of one's decisions at the time when this consumption is initiated.

APPENDIX 6A. THE RISK-PERCEPTION MODEL

The underpinnings of the analysis of the effect of age on risk beliefs can be seen using a Bayesian learning framework. In particular, we will use a beta distribution to characterize the learning process since this distribution is highly flexible and is ideally suited to analyzing binary lotteries such as this. Assuming a normal distribution yields an identical mathematical structure but imposes far more stringent symmetry requirements. This approach was introduced by Viscusi (1985) and Viscusi and O'Connor (1984). The formulation below introduces a variant of this model, recognizing three different sources of smoking risk information.

Individuals have three sources of information. First, they have their prior risk assessments p, which have associated informational content Ψ_0 (i.e., the informational weight placed on the prior is equivalent to observing Ψ_0 draws from a Bernoulli urn). The second source of information consists of direct and indirect individual experience. The individual may have been a cigarette smoker and formed a risk assessment based on the observed health effects (e.g., increased coughing), or one may learn about adverse health effects on others. Let q denote the risk assessment derived from experience, and γ_0 be the associated informational content. The third source of risk information consists of information about smoking that has been communicated to the individual, ranging from newspaper stories to hazard warnings on cigarette packages. Let r be the risk implied by this information and ξ_0 be its informational content. The final bit of notation is that it is useful to denote the fraction of the total informational content associated with each information source rather than its level, and we will drop the 0 subscript in this instance (i.e., $\Psi = \Psi_0/(\Psi_0 + \gamma_0 + \xi_0)$, $\gamma = \gamma_0/(\Psi_0 + \gamma_0 + \xi_0)$, and $\xi = \xi_0/(\Psi_0 + \gamma_0 + \xi_0)$.

The individual's lung cancer risk perception function takes the simple additive form,

$$\text{RISK} = \frac{\Psi_0 p + \gamma_0 q + \xi_0 r}{\Psi_0 + \gamma_0 + \xi_0} = \Psi p + \gamma q + \xi r, \qquad [6A.1]$$

so that the risk implied by each source of information is weighted by the fraction of the informational content associated with it.

The formulation in equation 6A.1 is particularly instructive in interpreting variations in risk perception with age and smoking status. The rows in Table 6–2 give lung cancer risk perceptions for different smoking groups, conditional on the age-group, and the columns give risk perceptions for different age-groups conditional on smoking status.

Suppose that publicly provided risk information conveys a higher risk than the individual's prior risk beliefs (r > p) and experiences (r > q). Even if the intent of the information campaign is to provide accurate information, limitations on individual processing of the information may lead to overassessments of the risk. As the risk perception literature has demonstrated, there is often a tendency for people to overassess highly publicized events.[19] Moreover, this coverage usually indicates that smoking is risky; it does not provide probabilistic information in any meaningful sense. If the saliency of the risk information creates a similar bias in the case of smoking, we would expect there to be overestimation of the risk. Other factors, such as the remoteness of the risk and the large size of the risk, may work in the opposite direction so that there is no unambiguous prediction from the risk perception literature pertaining to the direction of bias.

If, however, the sources of risk information have the associated probabilities indicated above, we would expect that as you move from the younger to the older age cohorts the risk perception should decline. For younger individuals the role of experience with cigarettes will be less, so that government information will play a greater role, leading to a higher risk assessment. The Bayesian learning model also predicts a dampening of the drop-off with age:

$$\frac{\delta^2 \text{RISK}}{\delta \xi_0^2} < 0 \text{ if p, q} < r.$$

This is in fact the pattern exhibited in Table 6–2.

APPENDIX 6B. THE ECONOMETRIC MODEL

The beta distribution formulation in equation 6A.1 leads quite directly to an empirical specification for purposes of estimation. The dependent variable in the risk perception equation pertains to lung cancer risks and not all risks of smoking. This equation provides only a partial assessment of the determinants of all smoking risk perceptions. The partial coverage creates no bias in the estimates for the determinants of lung cancer risk perceptions, since the lung cancer variable is the dependent variable in the analysis.

If we let X_{ji} be a vector of variables characterizing each source j of information for person i (i.e., j = 1 for prior beliefs, j = 2 for direct information transfer, and j = 3 for smoking-related experience), and let α_j be the associated vector of coefficients, then the lung cancer risk perception equation to be estimated for person i can be written

$$\text{RISK}_i = \alpha_0 + \alpha_1 X_{1i} + \alpha_2 X_{2i} + \alpha_3 X_{3i} + u_i, \qquad [6B.1]$$

where u_i is a random error term.[20] The variables included in X_{3i} include the respondent's past and current smoking status. Past smoking decisions are predetermined and consequently can be treated as exogenous. Current smoking status likewise may be predetermined because of the long-term nature of such consumption decisions, but on theoretical grounds current smoking status could be endogenous. Although one cannot reject the possibility that smoking status is not endogenous, I will also include results that allow for the possibility of simultaneity.

These estimators will also be used to assess the effect of the nonresponses to the RISK question. Table 6B–1 provides a comparison of the sample characteristics of individuals who responded to the survey and those who did not. For the most part, the composition of the samples is quite similar. The geographical distribution and smoking status of the nonrespondents closely parallel those in the full sample. The principal discrepancy is with respect to the age composition. Over two-thirds of the nonrespondents to the RISK question are age 46 or older, as compared with 37 percent overall. This pattern arises in other survey contexts where difficult or technical questions are being addressed, as older respondents often are less able to deal with these situations.

To test for the potential influence of selectivity bias with respect to the lung cancer risk responses, we will include the inverse of the Mill's ratio using a probit estimation procedure described by Heckman (1976). This hazard rate term pertaining to the probability of a nonresponse to the RISK question will be denoted by LAMBDA. One can consequently rewrite equation 6B.1 as

$$\begin{aligned}
\text{RISK}_i = {} & \alpha_0 + \alpha_1 X_{1i} + \alpha_2 X_{2i} + \alpha_3' X_{3i}' \\
& + \alpha_4 \text{ SMOKER}_i + \alpha_5 \text{ LAMBDA}_i + u_i \qquad [6B.2]
\end{aligned}$$

Table 6B–1 Characteristics of respondents who did not answer RISK question

Variable	Sample characteristics	
	Full sample Mean (std. dev.)	Nonrespondents to RISK question
AGE 16–21 (Age 16–21 d.v.)	0.113 (0.316)	0.037 (0.188)
AGE 22–45 (Age 22–45 d.v.)	0.512 (0.500)	0.255 (0.436)
AGE 46+ (Age 46 or older d.v.)	0.368 (0.482)	0.688 (0.464)
MALE	0.366 (0.482)	0.312 (0.464)
HOUSEHOLD SIZE	2.193 (0.983)	1.977 (1.009)
SMOKER	0.250 (0.433)	0.297 (0.457)
FORMER SMOKER	0.248 (0.432)	0.226 (0.419)
Northeast metro	0.170 (0.376)	0.176 (0.381)
Northeast nonmetro	0.042 (0.201)	0.026 (0.160)
North central metro	0.178 (0.382)	0.126 (0.332)
North central nonmetro	0.086 (0.280)	0.089 (0.285)
South metro	0.187 (0.390)	0.210 (0.408)
South nonmetro	0.129 (0.335)	0.167 (0.374)
West metro	0.169 (0.374)	0.171 (0.377)
West nonmetro	0.039 (0.195)	0.034 (0.182)
Sample size	3119	381

The dichotomous smoking decision is governed by the equation

$$\text{SMOKER}_i = \beta_0 + \beta_1 Y_{1i} + \beta_2 \text{RISK}_i + \epsilon_i, \qquad [6B.3]$$

where Y_{1i} is a vector of variables pertaining to tastes for cigarettes and cigarette prices. Because of the discrete nature of smoking status, equation 6B.3 will be estimated using probit analysis.

For the simultaneous equation estimation of equations 6B.2 and 6B.3, conventional two-stage least squares analysis is not appropriate because of the discrete nature of the smoking variable. Instead, I will adopt the procedure suggested by Maddala (1983, pp. 244–245). First, form the reduced form analogs of the risk perception and smoking probability equations.[21] The risk perception equation 6B.2 is then estimated by ordinary least squares after the SMOKER variable is replaced by the probit estimate of the smoking probability from the reduced form SMOKER equation. The smoking probability equation 6B.3 is estimated by probit after replacing RISK by the reduced form estimate of $RISK_i$. Appendix 6C discusses the estimator results.

APPENDIX 6C. TESTING FOR AGE DIFFERENCES IN SMOKING BEHAVIOR

To analyze smoking behavior, let the dependent variable be whether or not the individual smokes, which is a dichotomous 0–1 variable. The subsequent analysis of smoking behavior will consider the effect on smoking of a series of risk perception and personal characteristic variables. The first four equations in Table 6C–1 report the probit estimates of the smoking equation, where RISK is not treated as endogenous. The second set of equations at the bottom of Table 6C–1

Table 6C–1 Summary of teenager–risk perception interactions for probit estimation of smoking probability equation

	Coefficients (standard errors)		
Probit estimates	RISK	AGE16–21	AGE16–21 × RISK
Basic equation	−0.6716[a]	−0.4119[a]	0.2976
	(0.0999)	(0.1614)	(0.2976)
Basic ideas heard equation	−0.6872[a]	−0.4435[a]	0.3246
	(0.1004)	(0.1623)	(0.2982)
Basic and attitudes equation	−0.4992[a]	−0.3009	0.4811
	(0.1391)	(0.2112)	(0.3869)
Basic and ideas heard and attitudes equation	−0.5192[a]	−0.3383	0.0772
	(0.1402)	(0.2134)	(0.3887)
Simultaneous equation probit estimates			
Basic equation	−0.9998[a]	−0.3942[a]	0.3032
	(0.1289)	(0.1605)	(0.2965)
Basic and ideas heard equation	−1.0275[a]	−0.4271[a]	0.3339
	(0.1300)	(0.1614)	(0.2973)
Basic and attitudes equation	−0.6459[a]	−0.2608	0.0185
	(0.1812)	(0.2090)	(0.3831)
Basic and ideas heard and attitudes equation	−0.6776[a]	−0.2990	0.0131
	(0.1833)	(0.2113)	(0.3852)

[a]Denotes coefficients that are statistically significant at the 5 percent level, one-tailed test.

report the probit estimates obtained using the simultaneous model discussed in Appendix 6B.

Four different probit specifications are addressed in Table 6C–1. All equations include the lung cancer risk perception (RISK), whether the respondent is in the AGE16–21 age-group, and an interaction between AGE16–21 and RISK to identify a possible difference in smoking behavior. The basic equation includes these measures as well as three demographic variables and seven regional dummy variables. The second equation adds a series of four dummy variables for various ideas that the individual may have heard about smoking, such as that smoking is dangerous to one's health. These variables capture in part omitted aspects of risk information that may be pertinent to smoking behavior. The third specification adds a series of twenty-four smoking attitude 0–1 dummy variables. These variables are the results of an open-ended memory recall task in which the interviewer elicited the respondent's attitude toward smoking behavior. The overwhelming majority of the attitude probe responses were negative, as respondents indicated that smoking causes cancer, affects health, shortens life, or is otherwise unattractive. These memory recall variables capture tastes and omitted aspects of risk perceptions not reflected in the lung cancer variable.

The results are similar in each case. For each of the four specifications there is no statistically significant difference in the smoking behavior of the youngest age-group in the sample. The greater risk assessments of the AGE16–21 group are transmitted into reductions in smoking behavior in the same manner as for the rest of the population. In particular, the independent effect of the AGE16–21 coefficient and the interactive effect of AGE16–21 with RISK are consistently not statistically significant. Moreover, the independent influence of RISK indicates a significant negative effect of lung cancer risk perceptions on smoking behavior. These effects appear to be somewhat greater for the simultaneous equation model.

It should be noted, however, that the point estimates of AGE16–21 × RISK are always positive. Taken at face value, these results would imply that risk perceptions have a smaller effect for the young. Moreover, although none of the interactions are statistically different from zero, the point estimates of the effects are relatively large. Other analyses of the data, such as splitting the sample into separate age-groups, failed to identify any statistically significant effect of age on how risk perceptions alter smoking behavior. Other samples with a larger group of young respondents may, however, indicate differences that are not apparent in these data.

To assess the robustness of these smoking probability results, consider the logit results presented in Table 6C–2. The simultaneous model results are not included because of the specific dependence of the estimation procedure on the probit technique, but an instrumental variable estimator is used. Four different specifications are addressed in Table 6C–2. All equations include the lung cancer risk perception (RISK), whether the respondent is in the AGE16–21 age-group, and an interaction between AGE16–21 and RISK to identify a possible difference in smoking behavior. The equations follow the same pattern as those in Table 6–5 in

Table 6C–2 Summary of teenager–risk perception interactions for logit estimation of smoking probability equation[a]

	Coefficients (standard errors)		
Logit estimates	RISK	AGE16–21	AGE16–21 × RISK
Basic equation	−1.1169[b]	−0.3974	0.3606
	(0.1735)	(0.2976)	(0.5554)
Basic ideas heard	−1.1340[b]	−0.4535	0.3797
equation	(0.1744)	(0.2980)	(0.5554)
Basic and attitudes	−0.9005[b]	−0.0617	0.0550
equation	(0.2656)	(0.4235)	(0.7791)
Basic and ideas heard	−0.9241[b]	−0.1216	0.0767
and attitudes equation	(0.2674)	(0.4274)	(0.7824)
Logit estimates with RISK instrumental variables			
Basic equation	−0.9949[b]	0.1007	−0.7779
	(0.1986)	(0.3324)	(0.6714)
Basic and ideas heard	−1.0047[b]	−0.0587	−0.7904
equation	(0.1995)	(0.3332)	(0.6723)
Basic and attitudes	−0.7987[b]	0.4575	−1.1482
equation	(0.3088)	(0.4746)	(0.9598)
Basic and ideas heard	−0.8177[b]	0.4096	−1.1465
and attitudes equation	(0.3105)	(0.4784)	(0.9618)

[a] Each equation also includes a series of 7 regional dummy variables.

[b] Denotes coefficients that are statistically significant at the 5 percent level, one-tailed test.

terms of the variables included. The bottom panel in Table 6C–2 provides results in which the RISK variable is replaced by an instrumental variables estimator to partially control for a potential endogeneity and omitted variables bias in the measure of risk perceptions.[22] The estimates are quite similar using the reported RISK variable as with the instrumental variables estimator of it.

The results are nearly identical in each case. For each of the four specifications there is no statistically significant difference in the smoking behavior of the youngest members of the sample. The greater risk assessments of the AGE16–21 group are transmitted into reductions in smoking behavior in the same manner as for the rest of the population. In particular, the independent effect of the AGE16–21 coefficient and the interactive effect of AGE16–21 with RISK are consistently not statistically significant. Moreover, the independent influence of RISK indicates a significant negative effect of lung cancer risk perceptions on smoking behavior.

The magnitude of these impacts is also substantial. If, for example, all individuals believed that the lung cancer risk probability were .05, then the fraction of smokers in society would rise by .08.

NOTES

1. See U.S. Department of Health and Human Services (1988).

2. Also see Becker, Grossman, and Murphy (1990), Chaloupka (1990), and Stigler and Becker (1977).

3. Knight-Ridder news service, August 12, 1989, reprinted in *Durham Morning Herald*, p. 2A.

4. See Viscusi (1979).

5. See Becker, Grossman, and Murphy (1990), and Chaloupka (1990).

6. The highest motor vehicle fatality rate is for the 15- to 24-year-old age-group. See the National Safety Council (1988), p. 6. The role of teenage drinking and driving is explored in detail by Cook and Tauchen (1984). Blomquist (1988) overviews the role of alcohol consumption in models of auto safety.

7. National Safety Council (1990), p. 30.

8. The survey did not, however, determine whether children fully understand the health consequences of cancer.

9. For example, in the case of job safety, analysts have linked compensating differentials for risk with subjective and objective measures of risk, as in the case of Viscusi (1979) and Viscusi and O'Connor (1984), but these studies do not explore the perception bias issues in the same detail as is possible with the cigarette data. Studies of driving behavior and seat belt use, such as Arnould and Grabowski (1981), do not explore specific aspects of risk perceptions. Recent studies of hazard warnings, such as Viscusi and O'Connor (1984), Viscusi and Magat (1987), Smith et al. (1988), and Smith and Johnson (1988), do not explore the perceptional bias and behavioral response linkages to the same extent as they are examined in this paper. The study by Kunreuther et al. (1978) of disasters is also very extensive.

10. In 1979 male smoking rates were 3.2 percent (age 12–14), 13.5 percent (age 15–16), and 19.3 percent (age 17–18). Female smoking rates increase more steeply with age: 4.3 percent (age 12–14), 11.8 percent (age 15–16), and 26.2 percent (age 17–18). See U.S. Department of Health, Education, and Welfare, National Institute of Education (1979).

11. The difference in means for the AGE16–21 group minus AGE22–45 group and the associated 95 percent confidence intervals are the following: .063 ± .035 (current smokers), .039 ± .033 (former smokers), .057 ± .024 (nonsmokers), and .073 ± .016 (all respondents).

12. The difference in means and the associated 95 percent confidence levels for the AGE46+ group minus the AGE22–45 group are −.054 ± .026 (current smokers) and .001 ± .014 (all respondents).

13. The patterns for all age-groups combined are statistically significant. Most but not all of these differences for particular age-groups are statistically significant. The difference in RISK means and the associated 95 percent confidence interval for former smokers minus current smokers are −.016 ± .080 (AGE16–21), .008 ± .023 (AGE22–45), .093 ± .031 (AGE45+), and .040 ± .020 (all ages); for non-smokers minus current smokers the differences and 95 percent confidence intervals are .082 ± .041 (AGE16–21), .064 ± .022 (AGE22–45), .035 ± .025 (AGE45+), and .056 ± .016 (all ages).

14. For the sample of all individuals irrespective of smoking status, the difference in means and the associated 95 percent confidence interval is .064 ± .014, and for smokers it is .077 ± .032.

15. The survey results in Chapter 5 indicated that the overall assessed death risk from

smoking exceeds the assessed lung cancer risk and the actual mortality risk but by less than the ratio of the overall smoking mortality rate to the smoking lung cancer rate.

16. These variables represent different X'_{3i} values in equation 6B.2 in Appendix 6B.

17. Using the demographic variables and a set of fifty refined regional variables as instruments, one can estimate the instrumental variables for PAST SMOKER or SMOKER, which are included in addition to the variables in Table 6–4. This constructed variable had an estimated value of 0.0316 and a standard error of 0.0929, so that one cannot reject the hypothesis that the original PAST or CURRENT SMOKER variables are not endogenous. The smoking variable consequently passes the Hausman (1978) specification test. The excluded instrument set (i.e., the regional variables) also passes a test of overidentifying restrictions. Finally, making a distinction between past and current smokers was not consequential, as there was no statistically significant difference in the effects.

18. The instrument set was the same as was used to estimate the reduced form SMOKER equation. The CURRENT SMOKER variable has been jointly estimated using the two-stage procedure described above, and the PAST SMOKER variable is also an instrumental variables estimate.

19. See Camerer and Kunreuther (1989); Combs and Slovic (1979); Fischhoff et al. (1981); Lichtenstein et al. (1978); Viscusi (1985a,b, 1988), and Viscusi and Magat (1987).

20. The implications of estimating $\ln(1 + \text{RISK})$ are almost identical, but this formulation lacks the theoretical basis of the linear specification. Other nonlinear specifications of the risk-perception equation led to very similar results to those yielded by equation 2, so the analysis will focus on the simple linear model.

21. In each case I augment the set of instruments by fifty detailed regional dummy variables. Moreover, for the RISK equation I also include a variable for whether RISK was above or below its median in a procedure developed by Wald (1940) and described in Kmenta (1986, pp. 361–362).

22. In particular, the instruments used to construct the estimated value of RISK were a series of fifty regional dummy variables and 0–1 variable for whether RISK was above or below its median value. This two-stage least squares procedure is intended to reduce potential problems of bias.

7
The Quest for Rational
Risk-Taking Decisions

SMOKING BEHAVIOR AND ECONOMIC RATIONALITY

The primary intent of this investigation of smoking decisions has been to assess the degree to which this behavior is informed and obeys the properties of consistency that one would like to promote in any decision context. This assessment was based on detailed analysis of large bodies of empirical evidence, not on conjecture or anecdotal evidence.

We distinguished three different models that could be used to characterize this behavior. First, smoking decisions could be fully rational both in terms of the perceptions individuals have of the risk and in the extent to which they take these risks into account when making their decisions. Since a no-risk society is not attainable or even desirable, one might expect some individuals to rationally choose to smoke if the weight they place on the benefits derived from smoking exceeds their assessment of the expected loss stemming from the risks.

In a second framework, termed the "stylized smoker," individuals are viewed as being ignorant of the hazards they face; if they are aware of the risks, they ignore them when making their smoking decisions. It is this framework that is frequently used as the reference point in public discussions of smoking behavior.

The final model is that of a smoker with cognitive limitations. This individual does make smoking decisions based on risk information. However, the manner in which the risk information is processed and the character of the subsequent choices often reflect the anomalies and biases that have been identified in the substantial recent literature on economic behavior under uncertainty. There will, of course, be individuals of all three types in the population. The purpose of the empirical analysis has been to identify the most prevalent characterization of individual behavior.

Table 7-1 summarizes the implications of the empirical analysis for each of these three models. The first column in the table distinguishes the four different characteristics of behavior for which we will be making judgments. The second column of the table summarizes the empirical evidence that is pertinent to making judgments pertaining to each of these aspects of behavior, and the final column in Table 7-1 indicates the implications for each of the three different models of smoking behavior. In every situation one can reject the model of a

Table 7–1 Summary of research findings

	Empirical evidence	Implications for models of smoking behavior
Sources of information	1. Government, provision of information, particularly since 1964	1. Substantial information consistent with rational smoker
	2. Mandated cigarette warning labels, with the 1965 warning implying a lifetime cancer risk of about .12	2. Extensive risk information contrasts with stylized view of ignorant smoker
	3. Substantial media coverage of smoking risks, especially since 1960s	3. Highly publicized risks receive greatest prominence for smoker with cognitive limitations
	4. Prominence of smoking risks within smoking advertising since 1920s	
Risk perceptions	1. Public opinion poll trends indicate substantial and increasing awareness of risks and dramatic shift in willingness to restrict public smoking	1. Learning and age patterns consistent with rational smoker
	2. Perceived lifetime risk of lung cancer of .43 overall, .37 for smokers; "true risk" is .05–.10	2. Awareness of risks leads to rejection of stylized smoker model
	3. Much information about smoking risks has little effect on risk perceptions because of substantial information	3. Level of risk perceptions possibly too great for highly publicized lung cancer risks, consistent with model of smoker with cognitive limitations
	4. Depending on survey methodology, perceived lung cancer death risk ranges from .33 to same level as overall lung cancer risk	
	5. Total perceived smoking death risk is on the order of .59, or roughly two to four times the scientific estimates of total mortality risks	
	6. Younger age-groups (age 16–21) have higher risk perceptions since their mix of information is more recent	
Recognition of tradeoffs in decisions	1. Decline in smoking rates over time consistent with increased risk information and risk perceptions	1. Higher risk perceptions lower smoking rates, consistent with rational smoker; also consistency decisions in other risk contexts
	2. Negative mentions dominate responses to open-ended memory recall for cigarettes, indicating prominence of negative attributes	2. Tradeoffs inconsistent with stylized smoker
	3. Higher risk perceptions reduce smoking behavior; accurate lung cancer risk perceptions would raise societal smoking rates by 6.5 to 7.5 percent	3. Excessive risk perception as component of tradeoff consistent with model of smoker with cognitive limitations
	4. Cigarette demand declines with the price, consistent with patterns for normal economic goods; teenagers are most price-sensitive	

(continued)

Table 7–1 (*Continued*)

Empirical evidence	Implications for models of smoking behavior
5. Excise taxes endow individuals with a lung cancer risk-perception equivalent ranging from .17 to .51 depending on the elasticity of demand	
6. Smokers behave consistently in other risk-taking contexts, as they are willing to work on hazardous jobs for a lower amount of compensation per unit risk	
7. Younger age-groups (age 16–21) have the same smoking probability-risk tradeoff as their more senior counterparts	
Efficiency properties of smoking	1. Decisions are generally informed and reflect tradeoffs, consistent with efficient risk-taking behavior
	2. Stylized view of ignorant smoker who is unresponsive to economic incentives is rejected
	3. Possibly excessive response to risk aspect of decision due to substantial publicity; excess is much greater for lung cancer risks than for total risks of smoking; behavior consistent with observed decisions with respect to highly publicized risks

stylized smoker who is ignorant of the hazards posed by smoking and the importance of taking these risks into account when making decisions. There is much stronger support for the rational smoker framework and the model of smokers with cognitive limitations. The latter model is particularly pertinent with respect to the effect of extensive smoking risk publicity on smoking risk perceptions.

Let us consider each of the dimensions of the model in turn. The first component is the extent to which individuals have information concerning the risks. By almost any standard, smoking hazards are not hidden risks. For several decades, there has been substantial information provided through government reports by the Surgeon General and associated press releases, mandated hazard warnings and restrictions on cigarette advertising, media coverage of smoking risks, and mentions of smoking risks by cigarette companies within the context of cigarette advertising. Individual experiences of morbidity effects, such as shortness of breath, also provide the smoker with direct signals of other possible health-related effects of smoking.

The substantial information provided about the hazards of smoking is consistent with either the model of rational behavior or a model of smokers with cognitive limitations. There are, however, several characteristics of this information that are not conducive to a rational risk perception response. The substantial information provided need not lead to completely accurate risk assessments. Chief among the limiting factors is that this information typically does not indicate a smoking risk probability but instead simply indicates that smoking is harmful or has some probability of inflicting harm. In addition, individuals also receive information regarding total adverse outcomes linked to smoking (e.g., lung cancer death statistics), but there is seldom an attempt to provide information concerning the denominator of this calculation that would enable people to form a probabilistic judgment. Furthermore, the high public profile of the risk information serves to augment individuals' perception of the risk.

Perhaps the main feature of all this risk information is that its primary intent is to raise risk perceptions in a context where the assumed reference point is complete ignorance of the risk, whereas the more correctly defined objective of risk information is to achieve informed choice. The risks posed by smoking are not a certain outcome, notwithstanding official statements declaring that "smoking causes lung cancer." There is some probability between zero and one that such adverse effects will occur. There has been little effort to incorporate the probabilistic aspect of the risks into the risk information efforts, potentially fostering biased perceptions.

The assessment of the trends in levels of smoking risk perceptions indicates that awareness of smoking risks is substantial, as one would expect with a model of rational behavior. Awareness of smoking risks has become particularly great over the last half century. The active role of the government during the past three decades no doubt is an important contributor to the rise in risk awareness since the 1960s.

Overall, consumers believe that the risks of lung cancer posed by cigarettes are considerable. Indeed, their perception of the lung cancer risk from smoking dwarfs scientists' estimates of the actual risk level. This result occurs in part because lung cancer risk perception survey questions serve as a proxy for smoking risks more generally. Nevertheless, even the total perceived smoking mortality rate and the expected impact on life expectancy exceed scientific estimates of the adverse health effects associated with smoking. The extent of overestimation is less pronounced for the total mortality risk from smoking. This result reflects the greater prominence of lung cancer risks as compared with the other potential hazards of smoking.

Smoking risk perceptions that reflect an overestimate of the risk are consistent with patterns of individual response that have been observed more generally with respect to highly publicized risks. People tend to overestimate risks that are repeatedly called to their attention in terms of outcomes and body counts rather than specific probabilities or frequencies. Individuals believe the chance of being hit by lightning or struck by a tornado are much greater than they actually are because the publicity associated with these events is disproportionate to their frequency. This result contradicts the usual economic assumption that more information promotes more accurate risk information. Such a favorable result hinges upon an idealized form of information provision and individual processing of information that is not borne out in smokers' behavior.

The ultimate test of whether risk perceptions are of consequence is the extent to which they affect smoking decisions. One would expect a rational decision maker to respond to the risk in terms of making a risk-benefit tradeoff. There are several patterns of behavior that are consistent with such tradeoffs.

Smoking rates have declined over time, and there has been a change in the character of the product. Cigarettes now include lower tar and nicotine levels than before. Each of these developments is consistent with the greater value placed on risk over time as income levels have risen and as awareness of the risks has become heightened. The likelihood of smoking declines with the perceived lung cancer risk, and this response is quite substantial. Indeed, if smokers perceived the lung cancer risks from smoking as being comparable to what scientists estimate these risks to be rather than their current risk perceptions, societal smoking rates would rise by 6.5 to 7.5 percentage points.

Cigarette demand also declines with the price of cigarettes, as economists would predict, indicating a price tradeoff as well. This price mechanism takes on policy importance since it is the means by which excise taxes affect smoking. Cigarette excise taxes discourage smoking behavior in much the same way as would higher value-of-risk perceptions. The estimates in Chapter 5 indicate that depending on the assumed price sensitivity of cigarettes, excise taxes in effect endow individuals with a lung cancer risk perception for smoking of between .17 and .51. Thus, even if individuals were completely unaware of the risks of smoking, excise taxes would discourage smoking behavior by an amount that is not too dissimilar from the estimated total risks of smoking.

Ideally, we would also like to determine that these tradeoffs are not only substantial but consistent with other risk-taking decisions. Although refined judgments along these lines are not possible, there is broad evidence of consistency across classes of risk-taking behavior. Perhaps most noteworthy is that the wage-risk tradeoff rate displayed by smokers with respect to job risks is quite different than for nonsmokers. Indeed, the group most willing to bear job risks consists of those who smoke cigarettes and do not wear seat belts, which is the kind of pattern one would expect if risk taking were the result of a rational and consistent choice process.

The behavior of the young age-group is particularly important within the context of debates over smoking addiction. The evidence here runs directly counter to popular beliefs but in a manner consistent with rational learning models. Younger individuals are particularly likely to perceive the risks of smoking as being high because their mix of information about smoking is composed predominantly of recent data about substantial smoking risks. The effect of each unit of cigarette risk perceptions on the smoking rates is the same for the young as for older individuals. Coupled with the results pertaining to the overall high risk perception level on the part of the young, these findings strongly contradict the models of individuals being lured into smoking at an early age without any cognizance of the risks.

More generally, there is substantial evidence that individuals make tradeoffs with respect to smoking risks and other valued attributes. This behavior is consistent with both the models of rational behavior as well as other models that take into account the biases in decisions in contexts of uncertainty. Because of the inflated risk perceptions that are a component of these tradeoffs, it may be that the net effect is an overreaction to the risk, but the extent of any such bias is difficult to assess without a more precise reference point.

For much the same reason, making a distinction overall with respect to the efficiency of smoking is difficult. Ruling out the stylized smoker model is the easiest judgment to make based on these results. More refined judgments about the extent of the divergence from the fully rational outcome are difficult to make. However, the substantial risk overestimation and the evidence pertaining to smokers' tradeoffs between risk and other attributes of cigarettes suggest that it is unlikely that smoking rates greatly exceed what would prevail in a fully informed market context.

IMPLICATIONS FOR CURRENT SMOKING POLICY

The objective of smoking information policy should be to provide information so that individuals can make informed decisions. Ideally, we want individuals to have an appreciation of the diversity of potential risks posed by smoking as well as the consequences of these risks for their lives. After establishing this awareness of the risks, individuals then can use this information to make smoking decisions. An effort should be made to monitor this decision process to ensure that the tradeoffs are in fact reasonable, given the risk levels posed by cigarettes. Thus, the quest should be for informed and rational decisions, not necessarily a zero risk level.

If society wished to eliminate smoking risks, this goal could most readily be achieved by banning smoking altogether. We do not do this because we recognize that smoking offers other benefits to consumers. For much the same reason, we do not ban small cars, football, chain saws, scuba diving, bicycles, knives, sunbathing, and other risky products and activities that may offer some offsetting advantages.

In any economy there will be a broad range of tastes and preferences, and with this heterogeneity in tastes some people will place a greater value on risks. There will likewise be differences in the degree to which smoking is regarded as a pleasurable activity. The result of this heterogeneity is that smoking rates will differ, and people may quite legitimately differ about the attractiveness of smoking as a consumption activity.

However, the fact that most members of society currently choose not to smoke does not imply that the majority should impose their tastes on those who choose to smoke. The net financial externalities of smokers on the rest of society appear to be quite modest. The risks posed by secondhand smoke, which remain highly debated, can best be addressed by policies that directly limit the generation of this smoke in public places. The individual decision to smoke in contexts in which this risk will be borne by the smoker represents a potentially legitimate tradeoff that could rationally be made.

The government nevertheless does have a responsibility to ensure that these risk-taking decisions are in fact informed. The objective consequently should be to apprise people of the true risks posed by smoking and to enable them to make sensible decisions with respect to the risk.

This objective of effective risk communication is often confused with discouraging risky behavior. The policy intent should not be to simply raise risk perceptions to the highest possible level. Our purpose should not be to deter smoking but to provide information concerning the variety of smoking hazards, their magnitude, and their consequences for individual welfare. Thus, the policy objective should not be a smoke-free society but rather a society with informed risk-taking decisions. The result may be that once this informed-choice situation is achieved, smoking rates will decrease.

The antismoking policies that have been in place for the past several decades have bolstered risk perceptions and have led to a substantial reduction in smoking behavior. In terms of alerting consumers to the general risks of smoking, it appears that in many respects we have accomplished this goal. The potential hazards of smoking are not a closely guarded secret, and if anything risk perceptions for some smoking risks, such as lung cancer, may be too high.

A fundamental policy issue is whether we should continue our efforts to raise these risk perceptions even further. There is little question that overall smoking mortality risk perceptions are at least as great as the levels suggested by the scientific evidence. Any policy of risk information necessarily must reach some stopping point unless the risks posed are a certain outcome.

The science of risk communication is not nuclear physics. It is not feasible to communicate risks and precautions with total accuracy. Overall, perceptions of the total risks of smoking appear to be in the correct neighborhood and perhaps a bit high. From an informational standpoint, there is no rationale for boosting these perceptions even higher.

A frequent pitfall of informational regulations is that they do not serve truly informational objectives but instead are forms of persuasion. The government's experiences with informational regulations is replete with failures that attempted to browbeat consumers into changing their tastes. Policies of persuasion do not foster the objective of improving individual welfare given the diverse preferences of the citizenry. Not surprisingly, the policies that have attempted to alter choice rather than to inform decisions have not met with success. The risk-information efforts that have proven most effective are those that provide new knowledge in a clear and convincing manner. Smoking risk information policies have a legitimate role to play, but they must be guided by these principles for sound and responsible hazard communication.

Unfortunately, most policy proposals seek to do little more than intensify the current effort. There appears to be an ongoing quest for bolder warnings justified not by inadequate risk beliefs but simply by a desire to discourage smoking. The state of California introduced a vigorous antismoking advertising campaign in 1990, including messages such as "Warning: The tobacco industry is not your friend," and "Cigarette smoking kills more blacks than whites."[1] In 1991 the American Medical Association urged that the new warning for cigarettes read: "Smoking is ADDICTIVE and may result in DEATH."[2]

Intensifying the current hazard warnings poses several risks. First, excessive public efforts to raise risk beliefs may lead individuals to overassess the risks they face. What is at stake is not simply the legitimacy of a particular risk-communication policy but rather the credibility of the government's information-al efforts more generally. Smoking is not the only context in which the government provides information. Many government agencies provide consumers with risk information pertaining to the hazards posed by pesticides, pharmaceuticals, household chemicals, saccharin, and a variety of consumer products. If consumers come to believe that the government's informational efforts are designed to deter activities rather than inform decisions, then we risk having consumers dismiss the information. The government should never be placed in a situation of being an advocate against a legitimate activity but instead should take actions that are intended to assist individuals in making sound decisions.

Extensive public attention to one class of risks, such as those from smoking, also may distract consumers' attention from the other risks they face. Consumers' brains do not have an infinite storage capacity. They must necessarily be selective about what information they will acquire. The government in turn should attempt to select the contexts in which providing risk information can achieve the greatest gains in terms of moving people toward an efficient risk outcome. As I will indicate below, we can use this limited capability more effectively by changing the character of the smoking risk information provided. More can be done in the smoking information area, but the character of these efforts should be modified.

MARKET COMPETITION FOR SAFER CIGARETTES

Other smoking risk policies offer more promise than simply intensifying the current efforts. The typical regulatory strategy in other risk contexts is to foster technological solutions to safety. Mandated changes in technology, such as catalytic converters for autos and guards on machines, reduce the risks posed by the product. The introduction of filter cigarettes and the various "light" cigarettes are in the same vein. Companies altered the attributes of the product, reducing the estimated risk, but at some cost to other product attributes, such as taste.

The most dramatic technological change of this type was the introduction of the smokeless cigarette—Premier—by R. J. Reynolds. When R. J. Reynolds sought to enhance cigarette safety by introducing the Premier cigarette, for which there was no burning of tobacco, this product innovation was criticized by government officials. The Premier cigarette represented a substantial technologi-cal breakthrough in cigarette design. Rather than lighting tobacco, the consumer lit a carbon tip at the end of the cigarette, which otherwise had all of the external appearances of a conventional cigarette. This carbon tip in turn heated up an aluminum chamber filled with porous beads coated with tobacco extract. As these crystals vaporized, the smoke then passed through tobacco filters and through a conventional filter before being inhaled. There was no tobacco burned with this cigarette. There was some tobacco taste, but less than for conventional cigarettes. Smokers could continue to enjoy the sensation of smoking and the associated value they placed on nicotine, but the main valued attribute that Premier smokers lost was taste. In effect, this product simply pushed to the extreme the other cigarette safety innovations such as the introduction of filters and tobacco mixes with lower tar content.

Somewhat surprisingly, this technological change in cigarette design was the target of substantial criticism. Government officials attacked the Premier as a "nicotine delivery device." Whereas in other risk regulation contexts the government has mandated safety-related improvements, in the cigarette case it has actively discouraged the most important safety-related breakthrough in cigarette design.

The government's stance against the Premier cigarette is reminiscent of the 1960 position of the U.S. Surgeon General, who opposed the advertising that promoted low-tar cigarettes. This effort in turn led to a ban on tar and nicotine competitive advertising. Ironically, during the previous three years known as the great "tar derby," the cigarette industry achieved a one-third reduction in tar and nicotine through market competition.

In assessing the attractiveness of the Premier cigarette, it is best to conceptualize what this innovation meant to the character of cigarettes. Imagine that a cigarette had been developed that did not burn any tobacco and did not pose any risk of lung cancer. Carbon monoxide risks and risks such as heart disease would remain but would be no worse than with conventional cigarettes. The only other attributes of the cigarette that changed are the taste of the cigarette, which declined, and the fact that the cigarette had to be lit using a lighter rather than a match. In effect, this innovation simply carried to the extreme the types of changes that had been developing over the past two decades in terms of "lighter" filtered cigarettes with lower tar and nicotine. By eliminating burning tobacco and the hazards linked to it, the product simply altered the taste and potential hazards of cigarettes to a greater extent than any of the previous cigarette innovations. One can view this innovation as a technological breakthrough that pushed the "light" cigarette concept to the extreme.

R. J. Reynolds marketed this cigarette as offering "the cleaner smoke," an obvious reference to the risk attribute of cigarettes. Federal Trade Commission regulations prohibited R. J. Reynolds from advertising the Premier as being "safer" or making other health-related claims, even though a lower health risk was the key product attribute.

The brochure attached to the Premier cigarette pack described the main difference between Premier and conventional cigarettes:

> Premier is the first cigarette you smoke by *heating tobacco—not burning it.*
>
> It's a breakthrough that changes the very composition of cigarette smoke—substantially reducing many of the controversial compounds found in the smoke of tobacco-burning cigarettes. Those that remain include carbon monoxide, but the amount of carbon monoxide is no greater than in the best-selling "lights."
>
> What it all comes down to is a cleaner smoke—for you and everyone around you.[3]

Whereas the government fosters innovations of this type in other contexts, surprisingly government officials did not embrace this new cigarette design. Nicotine accompanied by the risks from burning tobacco was acceptable, but a product that eliminated many of these health risks became objectionable. The 1989 Report of the Surgeon General summarized the official anxiety over the marketing of the Premier and other such products:

> The marketing of a variety of alternative nicotine delivery systems has heightened concern within the public health community about the future of nicotine addiction. The most prominent development in this regard was the 1988 test marketing by a major cigarette producer of a nicotine delivery device having the external appearance of a cigarette and being promoted as "the cleaner smoke."[4]

This official concern was expressed despite the fact that Premier did not increase the nicotine level; it only dramatically reduced the *health* risks, particularly those related to cancer. Antismoking groups are reluctant to support safer cigarettes since they hope to eliminate smoking altogether by restricting the market to conventional, higher-risk cigarettes. Although perhaps well intended, this policy is not in the best interests of those whom we would like to protect. Suppressing comparative cigarette safety information and the development of safer cigarettes so as to discourage smoking in effect uses death as the principal deterrent to smoking. Smoking rates rather than health outcomes have become the major concern. A more appropriate policy for a democratic society is to promote informed consumer decisions from a variety of taste-risk options in the marketplace. Even if our sole objective were risk reduction, not consumer welfare, opposing the Premier cigarette in the 1980s and the low-tar cigarettes in the 1960s were not sensible policies.

The government also faces decisions with respect to other technological changes. Antismoking forces reacted similarly to the 1991 test marketing of the "de-nicotined" cigarette introduced by Philip Morris. These cigarettes contained approximately 0.1 milligrams of nicotine per cigarette, as compared with 0.9 milligrams for the Marlboro brand. Philip Morris test marketed the de-nicotined cigarette under the brand names Next, Merit Free, and Benson & Hedges De-Nic. Several antismoking groups criticized the company because of alleged health-related claims being made. Because nicotine does not affect cigarette flavor, these critics claimed that any mention of nicotine was necessarily a health claim. Antismoking groups petitioned the Food and Drug Administration, urging that nicotine be classified as a drug and regulated as such.[5]

The government policies now in place actively discourage safety innovations in cigarettes. At the same time, these officials continue to deplore the use of conventional cigarettes, with their far greater risks.

Somewhat paradoxically, the expected smoking risk resulting from the obstructionist policy position will be greater than if safer cigarettes are encouraged and consumers are given the information needed to properly assess their risks. These examples of inconsistent and, I believe, misdirected policy actions could have been averted if the government had a more principled basis for its policies that was grounded in advancing the welfare of consumers, recognizing the legitimate differences in preferences that may prevail.

The only instance in which paternalistic policies have a strong motivation is with respect to teenage smoking. Society limits a wide variety of decisions until ages such as 16 and 18. These restrictions pertain to voting in elections, dropping out of school, driving a car, drinking alcoholic beverages, joining the army, getting married, and seeing certain movies. In some cases these limits stem from a desire to prevent costs from being imposed on the rest of society. A teenager who drinks and drives poses a substantial threat, but a teenager who smokes cigarettes while driving does not. Nevertheless, there are some classes of choices that have major consequences, and for that reason society may wish to reserve the privilege of making these choices until a particular age is reached. These limits should, however, be set according to the age at which individuals are believed to be capable of making reasonable long-term decisions regarding their welfare, rather than some arbitrary date independent of the choice context. The emerging consensus of smoking restriction policies has focused age 18 as the minimum age for the purchase of cigarettes.[6] Based on findings in Chapter 6, this policy appears to run little risk of exposing uninformed decision makers to the potential hazards of smoking.

NEW OPPORTUNITIES FOR GOVERNMENT POLICY

One can also distinguish several legitimate, broadly based functions that the government should have. First, the government can either test cigarettes to determine their relative riskiness or develop standardized procedures for the companies to do so. In effect, the government could establish a scientific basis for enabling companies to determine the comparative merits of innovations in cigarette safety, such as the Premier cigarette and the de-nicotined cigarette, in a manner that will follow a standardized scientific norm.

Second, the government should establish a uniform warnings vocabulary for communicating the differing risk levels of cigarettes. At present, the informational thrust has been to emphasize the overall risks of smoking. However, efficient risk taking requires two things. First, consumers should know the overall risks associated with the product. In addition, they should be able to distinguish the differing levels of riskiness among different types of products. Advertisements giving tar and nicotine levels are a step in the right direction, but considerably more effort could be devoted to developing a systematic risk-communication framework for identifying the differing health implications that different brands of cigarettes may have.

The risk information currently provided is quite limited. Cigarette advertising must include information on tar and nicotine levels, but cigarette packages need not. This information provision also does not address other risks of cigarettes, such as levels of carbon monoxide, ammonia, or hydrogen cyanide. Although a detailed chemical breakdown of the constituents of tobacco smoke would inundate consumers with facts rather than inform them, there is a need for greater effort to communicate the various health-related dimensions on which cigarettes differ so as to promote market competition on these risk attributes.

Although individuals have good information about smoking risks overall, they know much less about distinctions between products. The extent of the information gap pertaining to risks across cigarette brands is reflected in the relative risk assessments of smokers.[7] In 1986, 50 percent of all smokers believed that all cigarettes are probably equally hazardous. Many other respondents gave vague assessments, such as saying they did not know the riskiness of their brand of cigarettes. The respondents who expressed some perception of risk differences consisted of 21 percent who believed that their cigarettes were less hazardous than others and 8 percent who believed that they were more hazardous.[8] Even for this small group there is no assurance that these beliefs reflect the actual relative riskiness of their cigarettes. An informational program that highlights these risk differences clearly would provide new information that would serve a constructive role.

The limited comparative risk information that respondents do have appears to be related to their cigarette brand choice. Individuals who smoke low-tar cigarettes ($\leq$ 3 mg. tar) are more likely to express concern about health risks of smoking (87.1 percent) than those in the highest-tar group ($\geq$ 21 mg. tar), for which roughly half (54.8 percent) express concern about the health risks.[9] Smokers appear to be making some effort to match their cigarette choices to their safety preferences. Better comparative risk information could enhance these efforts.

In addition to fostering safety innovations in cigarettes, the government also should continue to serve in its informational role. However, this effort should utilize scientific evidence pertaining to the implications of its risk communication efforts. In studies that my colleagues and I have undertaken for the U.S. Environmental Protection Agency, we have indicated how a government agency can develop more effective and accurate warnings through scientifically controlled studies that determine the degree to which we are informing consumers in the intended manner.[10] Unfortunately, there has been little controlled scientific evidence underlying the government's ventures into the cigarette warning arena. The U.S. Congress typically drafts its warnings by huddling together congressional staffers who are quite familiar with writing legislation but who have little expertise in hazard warnings. On occasion, hearings may be held and regulatory agencies may be consulted. In the case of the 1984 warnings, there was even an attempt to analogize to the cigarette warning case based on the results that had been found in the advertising literature concerning the novelty of the advertising message.[11]

These are steps in the right direction, but they fall far short of what is achievable in the context of effective warnings design. A more appropriate strategy would be to identify the diverse risks of cigarettes that we wish to communicate and to undertake experimental studies with different consumer groups to identify the most effective way to communicate this information in an accurate and convincing manner. The principal message of this study of responses to cigarette risk information is that the human cognitive processes are a critical intervening factor between the risk communication policy and the smoking policy outcome, not an incidental factor that one can take for granted. As in other hazard-communication contexts, care must be taken to ensure that the warnings strategy we have adopted will indeed be effective given these limitations on how individuals process risk information and make decisions under uncertainty.

Cigarettes are not the only context in which risk communication policies are flawed. In an earlier study, my colleagues and I found that some EPA-approved hazard warning labels for pesticides were excessively cluttered with risk information.[12] Consumers faced with cluttered labels perceived the products as being risky, but they had little notion as to what particular kinds of precautions to take. As a result, the overall effectiveness of such labels was quite low.

In the case of cigarettes, we have a somewhat different kind of distortion. Antismoking messages convey a sufficiently high risk to consumers. However, there is little effort to distinguish the comparative risks among different cigarettes and to provide incentives for safety innovation. In practice, consumers are faced with more than a decision to smoke or not smoke. The kind of cigarettes they smoke is also of consequence. In communicating the risk information pertaining to today's cigarettes, the government should provide comparative product information. In doing so, it should utilize scientific evidence that adjusts for the changing composition of the cigarette rather than relying upon studies that for the most part are based on the risk estimates pertinent to quite different cigarette products from an earlier era.

In the long run, there will be a rising consumer demand for safer cigarettes with fewer associated risks. As income levels increase and individuals place a greater weight on adverse health effects relative to other smoking attributes, the average risk posed by cigarettes will decline and smoking rates will decline as well. Decreased smoking of the current mix of cigarettes with their associated risks will be a natural development of the market that will occur as society becomes more affluent. Within the context of this shifting demand, government efforts that promote market competition for safety will lead to the reemergence of products such as the Premier cigarette that alter the attributes provided by the product to better accord with the changing preferences of smokers.

These market processes are quite powerful, and they are the same types of influences that have led to the dramatic decline in accident rates of all kinds throughout this century. If our objective is to further the well-being of our citizenry, the policy task should be to foster such changes by giving smokers adequate risk information. Doing so will also promote increases in the diversity of product choices, including new cigarette designs that pose a lower risk. Informed choices and the increased societal concern with health will generate a continued reduction in the health risks smoking imposes on our society. The promotion of more informed and responsible smoking choices should become our policy objective.

NOTES

1. "California Opens All-Out War on Tobacco and Its Marketing," *New York Times*, April 11, 1990, pp. A1, A12.

2. *Durham Morning Herald*, June 26, 1991, p. A12.

3. See R. J. Reynolds, Premier warning label, 1988.

4. U.S. Department of Health and Human Services (1989), p. 13.

5. *Wall Street Journal*, March 28, 1991, p. B8.

6. *New York Times*, December 11, 1989, p. C1.

7. U.S. Department of Health and Human Services (1989), p. 181.

8. An additional 13 percent believed that their cigarettes posed the same risk as others.

9. See Mulholland (1991). These results are based on data from the U.S. Public Health Service, the 1986 Adult Use of Tobacco Survey. Results for intermediate-tar groups appear more similar to one another

10. See, for example, Viscusi and Magat (1987).

11. See the Federal Trade Commission (1981).

12. See Magat, Viscusi, and Huber (1988), and Magat and Viscusi (1992).

Text of Survey Instrument
Used in Audits & Surveys Study

Respondent's Name: _____

City/State: _____

Telephone #: ( ) _____

AUDITS & SURVEYS, INC   PROJECT #4918
One Park Avenue   SEPTEMBER, 1985
New York, New York 10016

SMOKING STUDY

I am _____ of Audits & Surveys, a national survey research company. I am calling long distance and we are doing a study about cigarette smoking. In order to be fair, we need opinions from both smokers and nonsmokers. This will only take about 5 minutes.

A. How many people of 16 years of age or older currently reside in this household, regardless of whether they are at home now?

_____
NONE   TERMINATE

B. Read X'd phrase in appropriate group (based on answer to Q.A.)

1 Person
( ) Are you that person?
(If not, ask for that person)
Record Sex:
    Male ( )
    Female ( )

CONTINUE WITH INTERVIEW

2 People

( ) Is the older member of the household . . .
Male ( )
Female ( )

( ) Of these two people is the younger person . . .
Male ( )
Female ( )

3 People

( ) Is the oldest member of the household . . .
Male ( )
Female ( )

( ) Of these three people, 16 years of age or older, in terms of oldest, middle, youngest, is the person whose age falls in the *middle* . . .
Male ( )
Female ( )

( ) Of these three people is the youngest member . . .
Male ( )
Female ( )

4 or More

( ) Is the oldest member of the household . . .
Male ( )
Female ( )

( ) Is the next to the oldest member of the household . . .
Male ( )
Female ( )

( ) Of the people aged 16 or older is the next to the youngest . . .
Male ( )
Female ( )

( ) Of the people aged 16 or older is the youngest member . . .
Male ( )
Female ( )

1. When I mention cigarettes, what comes to your mind? PROBE: Anything else?

_____

_____

_____

2. Regardless of whether or not you agree, which of the following ideas have you heard about cigarette smoking? Have you heard . . .

	YES	NO
Cigarette smoking will most likely shorten a person's life	( )	( )
Cigarette smoking is dangerous to a person's health	( )	( )

Cigarette smoking is bad for a person's health, but not
dangerous   ( )   ( )

Cigarette smoking is not bad for a person's health   ( )   ( )

3. Among 100 cigarette smokers, how many of them do you think will get lung cancer because they smoke? (If "don't know," PROBE: "Just your best guess will do.")

_____

4. In which of the following categories do you fit? (READ LIST)

( ) A current smoker
( ) A former cigarette smoker
( ) Never smoked cigarettes

5. And finally, which of the following age groups are you in? (READ LIST)

( ) 16–21
( ) 22–45
( ) 46 or older
( ) REFUSED (Do Not Read)

Q. 1 "When I mention cigarettes, what comes to your mind?

Negative Health Effects (Net)

Causes Cancer (Subnet)

    Causes Lung Cancer

Causes Other Types of Cancer	Cancer of tongue, jaw cancer, mouth cancer, stomach cancer, prostate cancer
Causes Cancer (General)	DNDC in SUBNET 17½
Shortens Life, Kills	Can live longer if you don't smoke
Causes Other Diseases, Affects Health	Lung disease/problems, respiratory disorders/problems, affects breathing, shortness of breath, asthma, emphysema, bronchitis, heart disease/disorders, birth defects, harmful to pregnant women/fetuses, speeds up/changes metabolism, acts as a depressant, makes you weaker, affects physical activities, can't do as much, can't walk as far, can't work as hard, can't run, causes hypertension, poison, catch cold easily, hurts my throat, makes me cough, causes choking/coughing, makes me nauseous, upsets my stomach, gives me headaches, gets into/affects your skin, allergic to smoke
Addictive, Habit Forming, Like a Drug	Nicotine is a drug/narcotic, addictive, makes you want to smoke more, it's habit forming, like a drug

Know People Who Died or Got Diseases Because of Smoking	Husband/wife died from cancer/lung cancer, 3 brothers-in-law died from emphysema, father died from lung cancer due to cigarette smoking, always hear of people dying from smoking, uncle died from lung cancer and cigarette smoking had something to do with it
Polluting, Other Health Related Effects	Stains teeth, stains hands, irritates my eyes, makes my eyes water/burn, pollutes the air, don't like breathing in smoke, uncomfortable to nonsmokers
Bad, Dangerous to Health (General)	Unhealthy, dangerous to your health
Expensive, Costly	It's like burning money
Smokers Are Crazy/Idiots	Smokers are crazy/idiots/stupid/out of their minds
Trying/Have Tried to Quit	Trying to quit, would like to quit, should quit, tried to quit and couldn't
Have Quit, Used to Smoke	Used to smoke and quit, feel better/healthier since I quit
Hearing Cigarettes Makes Me Want One	
Never Want to Smoke	Never want to smoke, glad I don't smoke
Public Has Been Made Aware of Dangers to Health	Advertising/radio/TV says it's harmful to your health, everything I see/read or hear is against it, Surgeon General says it's bad for your health, package warns that it's dangerous to health
More Should Be Done to Discourage Smoking	Should stop advertising, take cigarettes off radio/TV, school children should be educated to the dangers of smoking, should stop making cigarettes, take cigarettes off market, stop subsidizing tobacco growers, package says it is dangerous to health yet government subsidizes farmers, government gets revenues from taxes
People Should Be Allowed to Make Own Choice	If they want to smoke that's their business/their problem, if they want to die that's their problem
Anything, Non-health Related Effects	Smells, smells up your clothes/house/furniture/hair/breath/skin, smelly/dirty ashtrays, smokers are rude/annoying/inconsiderate, don't like being subjected to it, it's offensive, can't tolerate people who smoke, it's dirty/disgusting, unattractive, won't allow in my home/car, should be banned in public places

Reasons for Smoking (All Mentions)

Relaxing, relieves tension, helps my mind function, helps release frustrations, calms me down, settles the stomach, like to smoke, enjoy smoking, like the taste/smell, smoke to keep from getting fat, prevents me from eating, need to do something when I drink, feel rotten till I have a cigarette

Skeptical, Don't Believe Smoking Harmful

Hasn't hurt me, don't believe it gives you cancer, not sure if it causes cancer, say it's harmful but I'm not sure, don't believe it's harmful, cigarettes have not done me any harm, does not affect me in any way, mother just died of cancer but never smoked, know people who have died of lung cancer and not smoked

Bibliography

Adler, R., and Pittle, D. (1984). "Cajolery or Command: Are Education Campaigns an Adequate Substitute for Regulation?" *Yale Journal on Regulation* 2: 159–194.

Akerlof, G., and Dickens, W. (1982). "The Economic Consequences of Cognitive Dissonance," *American Economic Review* 72: 307–319.

American Law Institute (1965). *Restatement (Second) of Torts*. St. Paul: American Law Institute.

Arnould, R., and Grabowski, H. (1981). "Auto Safety Regulation: An Analysis of Market Failure," *Bell Journal of Economics* 12: 27–48.

Arrow, K. J. (1974). "Limited Knowledge and Economic Analysis," *American Economic Review* 64: 1–10.

——— (1982). "Risk Perception in Psychology and Economics," *Economic Inquiry* 20: 1–9.

Atkinson, A. B., and Skegg, J. L. (1973). "Anti-Smoking Publicity and the Demand for Tobacco in the U.K.," *The Manchester School of Economics and Social Studies* 41(3): 265–282.

——— (1974) "Control of Smoking and the Price of Cigarettes: A Comment," *British Journal of Public Economics* 1(1): 45–48.

Baltagi, B. H., and Goel, R. K. (1987). "Quasi-Experimental Price Elasticities of Cigarette Demand and the Bootlegging Effect," *American Journal of Agricultural Economics* 69(4): 750–754.

Baltagi B. H., and Levin, D. (1986). "Estimating Dynamic Demand for Cigarettes Using Panel Data: The Effects of Bootlegging, Taxation and Advertising Reconsidered," *Review of Economics and Statistics* 68(1): 148–155.

Barzel, Y. (1976). "An Alternative Approach to the Analysis of Taxation," *Journal of Political Economy* 84(6): 1177–1197.

Baumol, W. J. (1986). "Productivity Growth, Convergence, and Welfare: What the Long-Run Data Show," *American Economic Review* 76(5): 1072–1085.

Baumol, W. J., and Bradford, D. F. (1970). "Optimal Departures from Marginal Cost Pricing," *American Economic Review* 60: 265–283.

Becker, G. S., and Murphy, K. M. (1988). "A Theory of Rational Addiction," *Journal of Political Economy* 96: 675–700.

Becker, G. S., Grossman, M., and Murphy, K. M. (1990). "An Empirical Analysis of Cigarette Addiction," National Bureau of Economic Research Working Paper no. 3322.

Bettman, J. R. (1979). *An Information Processing Theory of Consumer Choice*. Reading, Mass: Addison-Wesley.

Bishop, J. A., and Yoo, J. H. (1985). "Health Scare: Excise Taxes and Advertising Ban in the Cigarette Demand and Supply," *Southern Economic Journal* 52(2): 402–411.

Blomquist, G. (1979). "Value of Life Saving: Implications of Consumption Activity,"
    Journal of Political Economy 87: 540–558.
——— (1988). *The Regulation of Motor Vehicle Traffic Safety*. Boston: Kluwer Academic
    Publishers.
Brennan, T. (1989). "Helping Courts with Toxic Torts," *University of Pittsburgh Law
    Review* 51: 1–71.
Calfee, J. E. (1985). "Cigarette Advertising, Health Information and Regulation Before
    1970," FTC Working Paper no. 134.
——— (1986). "Cigarette Advertising, Health Information and Regulation," FTC Work-
    ing Paper.
——— (1986). "The Ghost of Cigarette Advertising Past," *Regulation* 10(6): 35–45.
Camerer, C., and Kunreuther, H. (1989). "Decision Processes for Low Probability Risks:
    Policy Implications," *Journal of Policy Analysis and Management* 8(4): 565–592.
Chaloupka, F. J. (1990). "Men, Women, and Addiction: The Case of Cigarette Smoking,"
    National Bureau of Economics Working Paper no. 3267.
——— (1991). "Rational Addictive Behavior and Cigarette Smoking," *Journal of Politi-
    cal Economy* 49(4): 722–742.
Comanor, W., and Wilson, T. A. (1974). *Advertising and Market Power*. Cambridge:
    Harvard University Press.
Combs, B., and Slovic, P. (1979). "Causes of Death: Biased Newspaper Coverage and
    Biased Judgments," *Journalism Quarterly* 56: 837–843.
Cook, P., and Tauchen, G. (1984). "The Effect of Minimum Drinking Age Legislation on
    Youthful Auto Fatalities, 1970–1977," *Journal of Legal Studies* 13: 169–190.
Crist, P. G., and Majoras, J. M. (1987). "The 'New' Wave in Smoking and Health
    Litigation: Is Anything Really So New?" *Tennessee Law Review* 54: 551–602.
Darby, M. R. (1984). "The U.S. Productivity Slow-Down: The Case of Statistical Myo-
    pia," *American Economic Review* 74: 301–322.
Eiser, J. R. (1983). "Smoking, Addiction, and Decision-Making," *International Review of
    Applied Psychology* 32: 11–28.
Eiser, J. R., and VanDer Pligt, J. (1986). "Smoking Cessation and Smokers' Perceptions
    of Their Addiction," *Journal of Social and Clinical Psychology* 4: 60–70.
Fischhoff, B., Lichtenstein, S., Slovic, P., Derby, S. L., and Keeney, R. L. (1981).
    Acceptable Risk. Cambridge: Cambridge University Press.
Fischhoff, B., and MacGregor, D. (1983). "Judged Lethality: How Much People Seem to
    Know Depends on How Much They Are Asked," *Risk Analysis* 3(4): 229–236.
Fuchs, V. R. (1986). *The Health Economy*. Cambridge: Harvard University Press.
Fujii, E. T. (1980). "The Demand for Cigarettes: Further Empirical Evidence and Its
    Implication for Public Policy," *Applied Economics* 12(4): 479–489.
Goodin, R. E. (1989). *No Smoking: The Ethical Issues*. Chicago: University of Chicago
    Press.
Gottsegen, J. J. (1940). *Tobacco: A Study of Its Consumption in the United States*. New
    York: Pitman.
Hadden, S. G. (1985). *Read the Label: Reducing Risk by Providing Information*. St. Paul:
    Westview.
Hamermesh, D. S., and Hamermesh, F. W. (1983). "Does Perception of Life Expectancy
    Reflect Health Knowledge?" *American Journal of Public Health* 73(8): 911–914.
Hamilton, J. (1972). "The Demand for Cigarettes: Advertising, the Health Scare, and the
    Cigarette Advertising Ban," *Review of Economics and Statistics* 54: 401–411.
Harris, J. E. (1980). "Taxing Tar and Nicotine," *American Economic Review* 70: 300–311.

Hausman, J. A. (1978). "Specification Tests in Econometrics," *Econometrica* 46: 1251–1271.

Heckman, J. (1976). "The Common Structure of Statistical Models of Truncation, Sample Selection, and Limited Dependent Variables and a Simple Estimator for Such Models," *Annals of Economic and Social Measurement* 5(4): 475–492.

Hersch, J., and Viscusi, W. K. (1990). "Cigarette Smoking, Seatbelt Use, and Difference in Wage-Risk Tradeoffs," *Journal of Human Resources* 25(2): 202–227.

Houthakker, H., and Taylor, L. D. (1970). *Consumer Demand in the United States: Analyses and Projections.* 2d ed. Cambridge: Harvard University Press.

Ippolito, P. M. (1987). "The Value of Life Saving: Lessons from the Cigarette Market," In Lester B. Lave, ed. *Risk Assessment and Management.* New York: Plenum Press.

Ippolito, P. M., and Ippolito, R. A. (1984). "Measuring the Value of Life Saving from Consumer Reactions to New Information," *Journal of Public Economics* 25: 53–81.

Ippolito, R. A., Murphy, R. D., and Sant, D. (1979). *Staff Report on Consumer Responses to Cigarette Health Information.* Washington, D.C.: Federal Trade Commission.

Johnson, P. R. (1984). *The Economics of the Tobacco Industry.* New York: Praeger.

Johnson, T. R. (1978). "Additional Evidence on the Effects of Alternative Taxes on Cigarette Prices," *Journal of Political Economy* 86(2): 325–328.

Kahneman, D., and Tversky, A. (1979). "Prospect Theory: An Analysis of Decision under Risk," *Econometrica* 47: 263–291.

Kahneman, D., Slovic, P., and Tversky, A., eds. (1982). *Judgment Under Uncertainty: Heuristics and Biases.* Cambridge: Cambridge University Press.

Kao, K., and Tremblay, V. J. (1988). "Cigarette 'Health Scare,' Excise Taxes, Advertising Ban: Comment," *Southern Economic Journal* 54(3): 770–776.

Keeler, E. B., and Cretin, S. (1983). "Discounting of Life-Saving and Nonmonetary Effects," *Management Science* 29(3): 300–306.

Keeler, T. E., Hu, T., and Barnett, P. G. (1991). "Taxation, Regulation, and Addiction: A Demand Function for Cigarettes Based on Time-Series Evidence," University of California, Berkeley, Department of Economics, Working Paper no. 91-173.

Kenkel, D. S. (1991). "Health Behavior, Health Knowledge, and Schooling," *Journal of Political Economy* 95(2): 287–305.

Kmenta, J. (1986). *Elements of Econometrics*, 2d ed. New York: Macmillan.

Koutsoyannis, A. P. (1963). "Demand Functions for Tobacco," *The Manchester School of Economics and Social Studies* 31(1): 1–20.

Kunreuther, H. (1976). "Limited Knowledge and Insurance Protection," *Public Policy* 24: 227–261.

Kunreuther, H., Ginsberg, H., Miller, L., Sagi, P., Slovic, P., Borkan, B., and Katz, N. (1978). *Disaster Insurance Protection: Public Policy Lessons* New York: Wiley.

Laughhunn, D. J., and Lyon, H. L. (1971). "The Feasibility of Tax Induced Price Increases as a Deterrent to Cigarette Consumption," *Journal of Business Administration* 3(1): 27–35.

Leu, R. E. (1984). "Anti-Smoking Publicity, Taxation, and the Demand for Cigarettes," *Journal of Health Economics* 3(1): 101–116.

Lewit, E. M., and Coate, D. (1982). "The Potential for Using Excise Taxes to Reduce Smoking," *Journal of Health Economics* 1(2): 121–145.

Lewit, E. M., Coate, D., and Grossman, M. (1981). "The Effects of Government Regulation on Teenage Smoking," *Journal of Law and Economics* 24(3): 545–569.

Lichtenstein, S., Slovic, P., Fischhoff, B., Layman, M., and Combs, B. (1978). "Judged Frequency of Lethal Events," *Journal of Experimental Psychology: Human Learning and Memory* 4: 551–578.

Lucas, R. E., Jr. (1986). "Adaptive Behavior and Economic Theory," *Journal of Business* 59(4), pt 2: S385-S400.

Lyon, H. L., and Simon, J. L. (1968). "Price Elasticity of Demand for Cigarettes in the United States," *American Journal of Agricultural Economics* 50(4): 888–895.

McAuliffe, R. (1988). "The FTC and the Effectiveness of Cigarette Advertising Regulations," *Journal of Public Policy and Marketing* 7: 49–64.

McGuinness, T., and Cowling, K. (1975). "Advertising and the Aggregate Demand for Cigarettes: A Reply," *European Economic Review* 6(3): 311–328.

Maddala, G. S. (1983). *Limited-Dependent and Qualitative Variables in Econometrics*. Cambridge: Cambridge University Press.

Magat, W. A., and Viscusi, W. K. (1992). *Informational Approaches to Regulation*. Cambridge: MIT Press.

Magat, W. A., Viscusi, W. K., and Huber, J. (1988). "Consumer Processing of Hazard Warning Information," *Journal of Risk and Uncertainty* 1(2): 201–232.

—— (1991). "Pricing Health Risks: Cancer and Nerve Disease," Report to the U.S. EPA and Duke University Working Paper.

Maier, F. H. (1955). "Consumer Demand for Cigarettes Estimated from State Data," *Journal of Farm Economics* 37(4): 690–704.

Manning, W. G., Keeler, E. B., Newhouse, J. P., Sloss, E. M. and Wasserman, J. (1989). "The Taxes of Sin: Do Smokers and Drinkers Pay Their Way?" *Journal of the American Medical Association* 261(11): 1604–1609.

—— (1991). *The Costs of Poor Health Habits*. Cambridge: Harvard University Press.

Marsh, A. (1985). "Smoking and Illness: What Smokers Really Believe," *Health Trends* 17: 7–12.

Mulholland, J. (1991). "Policy Issues Concerning the Promotion of Less Hazardous Cigarettes," Bureau of Economics, Federal Trade Commission, Working Paper.

Nader, R. (1972). *Unsafe at Any Speed*. New York: Grossman.

National Research Council (1986). *Environmental Tobacco Smoke: Measuring Exposures and Assessing Health Effects*. Washington, D.C.: National Academy Press.

National Safety Council (1988). *Accident Facts*. Washington, DC: U.S. Government Printing Office.

—— (1990). *Accident Facts*. Washington, DC: U.S. Government Printing Office.

Nichols, A. L., and Zeckhauser, R. J. (1986). "The Perils of Prudence: How Conservative Risk Assessments Distort Regulation," *Regulation* 10(2): 13–24.

Oster, G., Colditz, G. A., and Kelly, N. L. (1984). *The Economic Costs of Smoking and Benefits of Quitting*. Lexington, Mass.: D. C. Heath and Company.

Overholt, R. H., Neptune, W., and Ashraf, M. (1975). "Primary Cancer of the Lung," *Annals of Thoracic Surgery* 20: 511–519.

Payne, J. W. (1985). "The Psychology of Risk Taking," In G. Wright, ed., *Behavioral Decision Making*. New York: Plenum.

Peltzman, S. (1973). "An Evaluation of Consumer Protection Legislation: The 1962 Drug Amendments," *Journal of Political Economy* 81(5): 1049–1091.

—— (1975). "The Effects of Automobile Safety Regulations," *Journal of Political Economy* 83: 677–725.

—— (1987). "The Health Effects of Mandatory Prescriptions," *Journal of Law and Economics* 30(2): 207–238.

Peto, J. (1974). "Price and Consumption of Cigarettes: A Case for Intervention?" *British Journal of Preventive and Social Medicine* 28(4): 241–245.

Porter, R. H. (1986). "The Impact of Government Policy on the U.S. Cigarette Industry," In Pauline M. Ippolito and David T. Scheffman, eds., *Empirical Approaches to Consumer Protection Economics*. Washington, D.C.: Federal Trade Commission.

Pratt, J., Raiffa, H., and Schlaifer, R. (1975). *Introduction to Statistical Decision Theory*. New York: McGraw Hill.

Raiffa, H. (1968). *Decision Analysis*. Reading, Mass.: Addison-Wesley.

Randall, A., Hoehn, J. P., and Brookshire, D. S. (1983). "Contingent Valuation Surveys for Valuing Environmental Assets," *Natural Resources Journal* 23: 637–648.

Ringold, D. J. and Calfee, J. E. (1989). "The Informational Content of Cigarette Advertising: 1926–1986," *Journal of Public Policy and Management* 8: 1–23.

Russell, M. A. H. (1973). "Changes in Cigarette Price and Consumption by Men in Britain, 1946–71: A Preliminary Analysis," *British Journal of Preventive and Social Medicine* 27(1): 1–7.

Russo, G. (1987). "An Empirical Analysis of Cigarette and Physician Demand," University of Hawaii, Working Paper.

——— (1989). "An Optimal Cigarette Tax," Ph.D. diss., Northwestern University.

Schelling, T. C. (1984). *Choice and Consequence*. Cambridge: Harvard University Press.

——— (1986). "Economics and Cigarettes," *Preventive Medicine* 15: 549–560.

——— (1988). "Cigarette Smoking: A Study of Change in Behavior," Kennedy School of Government, Harvard University, Working Paper.

Schmalensee, R. (1972). *The Economics of Advertising*, Amsterdam: North-Holland.

Schnabel, M. (1972). "An Oligopoly Model of the Cigarette Industry," *Southern Economic Journal* 38(3): 325–335.

Schneider, F. W., and Vanmastrig, L. A. (1974). "Adolescent Preadolescent Differences in Beliefs and Attitudes About Cigarette Smoking," *Journal of Psychology* 87: 71–81.

Schneider, L., Klein, B., and Murphy, K. (1981). "Governmental Regulation of Cigarette Health Information," *Journal of Law and Economics* 24(3): 575–612.

Schoenberg, E. H. (1933). "The Demand Curve for Cigarettes," *Journal of Business* 6(1): 15–35.

Schuck, P. (1986). *Agent Orange on Trial: Mass Toxic Disasters in the Courts*. Cambridge: Harvard University Press.

Schwartz, A. (1989). "Views of Addiction and the Duty to Warn," *Virginia Law Review* 75: 509–560.

Shopland, D. R., Eyre, H. J., and Pechacek, T. F. (1991). "Smoking-Attributable Cancer Mortality in 1991: Is Lung Cancer Now the Leading Cause of Death Among Smokers in the United States," *Journal of the National Cancer Institute* 83(16): 1142–1148.

Shoven, J. B., Sundberg, J. O., and Bunker, J. P. (1987). "The Social Security Cost of Smoking," National Bureau of Economic Research Working Paper no. 2234.

Slovic, P., Fischhoff, B., and Lichtenstein, S. (1979). "Rating the Risks," *Environment* 21(3): 14–39.

——— (1980a). "Facts and Fears: Understanding Perceived Risk," In R. Shwing and W. A. Albers, eds., *Societal Risk Assessment: How Safe is Safe Enough?* New York: Plenum.

——— (1980b). "Informing People About Risk," In L. A. Morris, M. Mazis, and I. Barofsky, eds., *Product Labeling and Health Risks*. Cold Spring Harbor, N.Y.: Cold Spring Harbor Laboratory.

Smith, V. K., and Johnson, F. R. (1988). "How Do Risk Perceptions Respond to Information? The Case of Radon," *Review of Economics and Statistics* 70: 1–8.

Smith, V. K., Desvousges, W., Fisher, A., and Johnson, F. R. (1988). "Learning about Radon's Risk," *Journal of Risk and Uncertainty* 1(2): 233–258.

Smith, V. K., Desvousges, W., Johnson, F. R., and Fisher, A. (1990). "Can Public Information Programs Affect Risk Perceptions?" *Journal of Policy Analysis and Management* 9(1): 41–59.

Staelin, R. (1978). "The Effects of Consumer Education on Consumer Product Safety Behavior," *Journal of Consumer Research* 5: 30–40.

Stigler, G. J., and Becker, G. S. (1977). "De Gustibus non Est Disputandum," *American Economic Review* 67(2): 76–90.

Stone, R. (1954). *The Measurement of Consumers' Expenditures and Behavior in the United Kingdom, 1920–1938.* Vol. 1. Cambridge: Cambridge University Press.

Sullivan, D. (1985). "Testing Hypotheses about Firm Behavior in the Cigarette Industry," *Journal of Political Economy* 93(3): 586–598.

Sumner, D. A., and Alston, J. (1984). "Effects of the Tobacco Program: An Analysis of Deregulation," American Enterprise Institute Occasional Paper no. 1–71.

Sumner, M. T. (1971). "The Demand for Tobacco in the U. K.," *The Manchester School of Economics and Social Studies* 39(1): 23–36.

Svenson, O. (1979). "Are We All among the Better Drivers?" Unpublished manuscript, Department of Psychology, University of Stockholm.

Tate, C. (1989). "In the 1800's, Antismoking Was a Burning Issue," *Smithsonian* 20(4): 107–109.

Tennant, R.B. (1950). *The American Cigarette Industry: A Study in Economic Analysis and Public Policy.* New Haven: Yale University Press.

Thaler, R., and Rosen, S. (1976). "The Value of Saving a Life: Evidence from the Labor Market," In N. Terleckyj, ed., *Household Production and Consumption.* New York: Columbia University Press.

Tobacco Institute (1987). *The Tax Burden on Tobacco: Historical Compilation 1986.* Vol. 21. Washington, D.C.: Tobacco Institute.

——— (1989). *The Tax Burden on Tobacco: Historical Compilation 1988.* Vol. 23. Washington, D.C.: Tobacco Institute.

——— (1990). *The Tax Burden on Tobacco: Historical Compilation 1989.* Vol. 24. Washington, D.C.: Tobacco Institute.

———, (1991). *The Tax Burden on Tobacco: Historical Compilation 1990.* Vol. 25 Washington, D.C.: Tobacco Institute.

Tollison, R. D., and Wagner, R. E. (1988). *Smoking and the State: Social Costs, Rent Seeking, and Public Policy.* Lexington, Mass.: D.C. Heath and Company.

Travis, C., Richter, S. A., Crouch, E. A. C., Wilson, R., and Klema, E. D. (1987). "Cancer Risk Management: A Review of 132 Federal Regulatory Decisions," *Environmental Science Technology* 21: 415–420.

Tversky, A., and Kahneman, D. (1981). "The Framing of Decisions and the Psychology of Choice," *Science* 211: 453–458.

——— (1982). "Judgment under Uncertainty: Heuristics and Biases," In D. Kahneman, P. Slovic, and A. Tversky, eds., *Judgment under Uncertainty: Heuristics and Biases.* Cambridge: Cambridge University Press.

U.S. Department of Commerce, Bureau of the Census (1966). *Statistical Abstract of the United States: 1966.* 87 ed. Washington, D.C.: U.S. Government Printing Office.

——— (1985). *Statistical Abstract of the United States: 1986.* 106th ed. Washington, D.C.: U.S. Government Printing Office.

—— (1989). *Statistical Abstract of the United States: 1989*. 109th ed. Washington, D.C.: U.S. Government Printing Office.

U. S. Department of Health, Education and Welfare (1964). *Smoking and Health: Report of the Advisory Committee to the Surgeon General of the Public Health Service*. Princeton: Van Nostrand.

—— (1967). *The Health Consequences of Smoking: A Public Health Service Review*, A report of the Surgeon General. Washington, D.C.: U.S. Government Printing Office.

—— (1968). *Supplement to the 1967 Public Health Service Review*, A report of the Surgeon General. Washington, D.C.: U.S. Government Printing Office.

—— (1969). *Supplement to the 1967 Public Health Service Review*, A report of the Surgeon General. Washington, D.C.: U.S. Government Printing Office.

—— (1971). *The Health Consequences of Smoking*, A report of the Surgeon General. Washington, D.C: U.S. Government Printing Office.

—— (1972). *The Health Consequences of Smoking*, A report of the Surgeon General. Washington, D.C.: U.S. Government Printing Office.

—— (1973). *The Health Consequences of Smoking*, A report of the Surgeon General. Washington, D.C.: U.S. Government Printing Office.

—— (1974). *The Health Consequences of Smoking*, A report of the Surgeon General. Washington, D.C.: U.S. Government Printing Office.

—— (1975). *The Health Consequences of Smoking*, A report of the Surgeon General. Washington, D.C.: U.S. Government Printing Office.

—— (1976). *The Health Consequences of Smoking: Selected Chapters from the 1971– 1975 Reports*, A report of the Surgeon General. Washington, D.C.: U.S. Government Printing Office.

—— (1977–1978). *The Health Consequences of Smoking*, A report of the Surgeon General. Washington, D.C.: U.S. Government Printing Office.

—— (1979). *Smoking and Health: The Health Consequences of Smoking, The Behavioral Aspects of Smoking, Education and Prevention*, A report of the Surgeon General. Washington, D.C.: U.S. Government Printing Office.

U.S. Department of Health, Education, and Welfare, National Institute of Education, (1979). *Teenage Smoking: Immediate and Long-term Patterns*. Washington, D.C.: U.S. Government Printing Office.

U.S. Department of Health and Human Services (1980). *The Health Consequences of Smoking for Women*, A report of the Surgion General. Washington, D.C.: U.S. Government Printing Office.

—— (1981). *The Health Consequences of Smoking: The Changing Cigarette*, A report of the Surgeon General. Washington, D.C.: U.S. Government Printing Office.

—— (1982). *The Health Consequences of Smoking: Cancer*, A report of the Surgeon General. Washington, D.C.: U.S. Government Printing Office.

—— (1983). *The Health Consequences of Smoking: Cardiovascular Disease*, A report of the Surgeon General. Washington, D.C.: U.S. Government Printing Office.

—— (1984). *The Health Consequences of Smoking: Chronic Obstructive Lung Disease*, A report of the Surgeon General. Washington, D.C.: U.S. Government Printing Office.

—— (1985). *The Health Consequences of Smoking: Cancer and Chronic Lung Disease in the Workplace*, A report of the Surgeon General. Washington, D.C.: U.S. Government Printing Office.

—— (1986). *The Health Consequences of Involuntary Smoking*, A report of the Surgeon General. Washington, D.C.: U.S. Government Printing Office.

———— (1988). *The Health Consequences of Smoking: Nicotine Addiction*, A report of the Surgeon General. Washington: U.S. Government Printing Office.

———— (1989). *Reducing the Health Consequences of Smoking: 25 Years of Progress*, A report of the Surgeon General. Washington, D.C.: U.S. Government Printing Office.

———— (1990). *The Health Benefits of Smoking Cessation*, A report of the Surgeon General. Washington, D.C.: U.S. Government Printing Office.

U.S. Federal Trade Commission (May 1981). Staff Report on the Cigarette Advertising Investigation, Washington, D.C.

Vernon, J., Rives, N. W., and Naylor, T. H. (1969). "An Econometric Model of the Tobacco Industry," *Review of Economics and Statistics* 61: 149–158.

Viscusi, W. K. (1979). *Employment Hazards: An Investigation of Market Performance*. Cambridge: Harvard University Press.

———— (1983). *Risk by Choice: Regulating Health and Safety in the Workplace*. Cambridge: Harvard University Press.

———— (1984). *Regulating Consumer Product Safety*. Washington, D.C.: American Enterprise Institute.

———— (1985a). "A Bayesian Perspective on Biases in Risk Perception," *Economic Letters* 17: 59–62.

———— (1985b). "Are Individuals Bayesian Decision Makers?" *American Economic Review* 75(2): 381–385.

———— (1986). "The Valuation of Risks to Life and Health: Guidelines for Policy Analysis," In J. Bentkover, V. Covello, and J. Mumpower, eds., *Benefit Assessment: The State of Art*. Dordrecht: Reidel Publishers, pp. 193–210.

———— (1988). "Predicting the Effects of Food Cancer Warnings on Consumers," *Food Drug Cosmetic Law Journal* 42: 283–307.

———— (1989a). "Prospective Reference Theory: Toward an Explanation of the Paradoxes," *Journal of Risk and Uncertainty* 2(3): 235–264.

———— (1989b). "The Political Economy of Risk Communication Policies for Consumer Products," In J. Shogren, ed., *Perspectives on Government Regulation*. Boston: Kluwer Academic Publishers, 83–129.

———— (1990a). "Do Smokers Underestimate Risks?" *Journal of Political Economy* 98(6): 1253–1269.

———— (1990b). "Sources of Inconsistency in Societal Responses to Health Risks," *American Economic Review* 80(2): 257–261.

———— (1991a). "Age Variations in Risk Perceptions and Smoking Decisions," *Review of Economics and Statistics* 73: 577–588.

———— (1991b). *Reforming Products Liability*. Cambridge: Harvard University Press.

———— (1992). "The Mis-Specified Agenda: Health, Safety and Environmental Regulation in the 1980's," In Martin Feldstein, ed., *American Economic Policy in the 1980's*. National Bureau of Economic Research, forthcoming.

Viscusi, W. K., and Evans, W. (1990). "Utility Functions That Depend on Health Status: Estimates and Economic Implications," *American Economic Review* 80(3): 353–374.

Viscusi, W. K., and Magat, W. A. (1987). *Learning about Risk: Consumer and Worker Responses to Hazard Information*. Cambridge: Harvard University Press.

———— (1989). "Right to Know and Behavioral Responses to Hazard Warnings," In Lester B. Lave, ed., *Risk Assessment and Management*. New York: Plenum Press, 70–89.

Viscusi, W. K., Magat, W. A., and Huber, J. (1987). "An Investigation of the Rationality of Consumer Valuations of Multiple Health Risks," *Rand Journal of Economics* 18(4): 465–479.

——— (1988). "Consumer Processing of Hazard Warning Information," *Journal of Risk and Uncertainty*, 1(2): 201–232.

——— (1992). "Communication of Ambiguous Risk Information," In John Geweke, ed., *Conference Volume for the Fifth International Conference on the Foundation and Application of Utility, Risk, and Decision Theories*. Boston: Kluwer Academic Publishers, forthcoming; also *Theory and Decision*, forthcoming.

Viscusi, W. K., and O'Connor, C. (1984). "Adaptive Responses to Chemical Labeling: Are Workers Bayesian Decision Makers?" *American Economic Review* 74(5): 942–956.

Wald, A. (1940). "The Fitting of Straight Lines if Both Variables Are Subject to Errors," *Annals of Mathematical Statistics* 11: 284–300.

Warner, K. E. (1977). "The Effects of the Anti-Smoking Campaign on Cigarette Consumption," *American Journal of Public Health* 67(7): 645–650.

——— (1981). "Cigarette Smoking in the 1970's: The Impact of the Antismoking Campaign," *Science* 211(4483): 729–731.

——— (1986). *Selling Smoke: Cigarette Advertising and Public Health*. Washington, D.C.: American Public Health Association.

——— (1989). "Effects of the Antismoking Campaign: An Update," *American Journal of Public Health* 79(2): 144–151.

Wasserman, J., Manning, W. G., Newhouse, J. P., and J. D. Winkler (1991). "The Effects of Excise Taxes and Regulations on Cigarette Smoking," *Journal of Health Economics* 10(1): 43–64.

Wildavsky, A. (1988). *Searching for Safety*. New Brunswick: Transaction Publishers.

Witt, S. F., and Pass, C. L. (1981). "The Effects of Health Warnings and Advertising on the Demand for Cigarettes," *Scottish Journal of Political Economy* 28(1): 86–91.

——— (1983). "Forecasting Cigarette Consumption: The Casual Model Approach," *International Journal of Social Economics* 10(3): 18–33.

Young, T. (1983). "The Demand for Cigarettes: Alternative Specifications of Fujii's Model," *Applied Economics* 15(2): 203–211.

Zeckhauser, R. J., and Viscusi, W. K. (1990). "Risk Within Reason," *Science* 248(4955): 559–564.

Index